Dr. Mary Beth Engrav

Stories from the Emergency Department

ISBN: 1-4565-7068-4
ISBN-13: 9781456570682

I have worked in a busy Emergency Department for 20 years. The Emergency Department is not a microcosm of life. It is a giant, blown up, dramatic picture of life at every extreme.

If I saw many of the situations I have taken care of on TV I would say that they never could have happened, they must be made up. In the Emergency Department every day I see things that I have never seen before, even in 20 years of practice.

Every day we work with patients who are often having the worst day of their lives, and our only job is to try to help them in any way we can. It can lead to some interesting situations that I will never forget. I feel grateful to be able to help patients on what is one of the worst day of their lives.

All of the stories in this book are true, but some details and all names have been changed.

Lacerations

On an average shift as an Emergency Physician, I usually repair three or four lacerations a night. I typically enjoy repairing cuts. Most Emergency Physicians enjoy procedures, and suturing is the most common of any of the procedures performed in the Emergency Department.

Very often, I would estimate 75% of the time, the patient who needs suturing is a child. Children manage to cut themselves in an amazing variety of ways. The most common of course is striking their head on a coffee table. I have often thought that all coffee tables should be banned from the home until children are six or seven. Children also often strike their heads on counters, fall/get pushed off bunk beds, fall off bikes/scooters/skateboards; there are a million different things active children can do to cut themselves.

Once I even took care of a child who managed to cut his head open in an inflatable "Joy Jump", when he was the only one in it. How you can cut your head in an inflatable, padded room is amazing to me.

I have had parents who go to extreme measures to child proof their house, and their kids still get hurt. I had a child who fell into a coffee table that had been covered with padding from one of those companies that childproof your house, and the child still got a huge forehead laceration. The dad was amazed as was I. He told me how they had hired the company to come in and child-proof every inch of their house, and this still happened.

For a child, having a laceration and then being taken to an Emergency Department is a truly horrifying event. Trying to gain the child's trust and getting them through the experience is a real challenge, but to tell the truth I enjoy it a great deal. I enjoy meeting the child initially, trying to gain their trust, and reassuring them that we will take care of them and they will soon be home.

It starts when you walk in the room. You have to initially assess the age of the child and the interactions with the parents, and depending on your feeling for the situation, start talking to the family or the child. I often address mainly the child with explanations later to the family, especially if the child is older.

Of course, if the child is less than 18 months all bets are off. A small cut under this age is best just taken care of expediently as possible by gently wrapping the child in a sheet, holding them still, numbing it up and repairing it. They simply cannot be talked through the procedure under 18 months, in my experience. It is simply a matter of getting it over with.

I have had a few parents demand sedative medication for their child at this age; and I will give it if they really want it and understand the risks. My personal opinion is that the risks of sedatives outweigh the benefits if it is a small laceration that I can repair in less than 10 minutes. Sedatives typically require an IV, which is painful, monitoring for hours afterwards, and of course the biggest risk, respiratory depression. Not really worth it for a 10 minute procedure in my opinion. We numb the wound with topical and then injectable medication so they child won't have pain. They still usually scream because they don't want to be held down; completely understandable as a toddler.

One child I will always remember was an 8-year-old with a two centimeter forehead laceration. She had been playing with her sister and struck her head on the counter in the kitchen. She was tiny with a blond ponytail and holding a stuffed bear. She was quite calm when I walked in the room with her chart, but I could see in her eyes that she was very nervous. After talking with her and explaining to her we would need to repair it, and that we could give her a topical pain medication, I saw two giant tears form in her eyes, but she was trying not to cry. It broke my heart on the spot. I reassured her again, as the nurse went to get the topical medication. Her mother comforted her, assuring her that it would be over soon.

We leave the topical medication on for about 15 minutes, and during that time I was off seeing other patients. My technician had a tray set up for me with injectable lidocaine, should I need it, and suture materials.

When I walked back in the room, I struck up a conversation with her that continued as I begun my work. Fortunately, the topical pain medication was completely successful. I washed the wound carefully and explored it. She had no pain. She was chatting happily now. I slightly touched the edge of the wound with the suturing needle and asked if she had pain. "No! I can't feel anything!" she said, completely shocked. I began my repair. I asked her about her family, and she told me she had a one year old little sister. I asked what types of things her sister likes to do, "she just likes to run around and dance", she said sweetly. She proceeded to tell me all about her sister, their pet dog, and what they had done that summer. What a happy, great kid.

After I was finished, she was quite proud of herself, as was mom, that she made it through the entire repair without crying. It went quickly, and we gave her a small stuffed animal and discharged her.

Several weeks later, I received a hand-addressed envelope in my mailbox when I went in for a night shift. In it was a hand-made thank you card, where she had drawn small broken hearts, then had drawn hearts that had been "stitched up". Thanks for fixing me", it stated in her handwriting, and she had signed her name. I still have that card in my mailbox, every now and then I look at it, especially before night shifts. She is a good example of why I love taking care of kids.

Another child who stands out, for different reasons, was a three-year-old with a scalp laceration who I will call Max. Max was there with his mother who seemed even more unhappy than the average parent to be at the Emergency Department. Max had, of course, hit his head on the coffee table, the bane of a three-year-old's existence. He had a very small, approximately 1 centimeter laceration, but it needed stitches.

At this age, I would estimate that 90% of the time I can reason with the child, have a long discussion about imaginary things and fairy tales that I make up, and we get them through it. One of my go-to-stories is about Sam, the baby elephant at our zoo, who most kids have seen. We talk about the baby elephant, what he eats, how he eats with his trunk, his mom, etc.

By age two to three I pride myself on making the Emergency Department a good experience for the child, or at least not a bad experience, by engaging them and developing a relationship with them. Right away, I realized that may not be the case with young Max. He was screaming with any attempt to just look at the laceration, even though I didn't even touch him. By the time he had seen three of us in our dark blue scrubs (the triage nurse, the nurse, and me), he would scream even if he saw someone walk by in the hallway in scrubs. Kids are amazingly smart like that.

We decided it would be in his best interest to restrain him in a sheet which we gently wrap around the child; it is less traumatizing than the old boards with Velcro straps we used to use. His mother agreed. We gave him a small dose of sedative medicine as he was so remarkably agitated, part of which he spit back at the nurse. He ripped off his topical medication and screamed bloody murder even when the nurse had tried to apply it.

After he was held down gently, I began to numb the wound with injectable lidocaine. Prior to that, I was just looking at the wound to assess it, and during that brief minute he started screaming like crazy. If a child is screaming even when we aren't doing anything yet, even though they've received the topical numbing which works very well, I can't gauge their pain response during the procedure. So I just have to go ahead and put injectable numbing medicine into the laceration to be sure I'm not hurting them while stitching.

"JESUS FUCKING CHRIST!" I thought he screamed as I carefully injected his laceration. I shook my head slightly, and thought to myself, I'm sure I misunderstood what he just said. Sometimes when kids are crying you can almost hear words in the cry. I started washing the wound. "FUCK! FUCK!' he yelled. Everyone in the department was now quite silent, as they could hear this. As we continued, we were treated to every bad word in the English language. From a three-year-old? Could this be right? I glanced quickly at the mother as I worked, she had her hands on his legs, helping hold Max, and her head was down. She was doing deep breathing exercises, the kind you do during labor.

As we wrapped up, after about 10 minutes of suturing, I pretended I hadn't heard anything and started giving her wound-care instructions as the technician cleaned the wound and lifted Max up out of the sheet.

"I want to tell you, I really apologize for the language. He has four older brothers, the oldest is 17, and he has really learned all of the words and when to use it," she said.

This made it quite understandable to all of us, and we all got a laugh out of it. When I think about it, he was just saying what every toddler who is sutured would like to tell us but can't. Needless to say, I did not receive a thank you card from Max or his mother, but I still think about him often.

Parents are almost always helpful during these procedures. The only time I have a real problem with parents is when they keep repeating things like "does it hurt you?" "are you in pain?" over and over again. Kids are amazingly suggestible, and if we have given them topical numbing, then deep numbing, and I have explained that to the parent, and the kid doesn't complain when I test the area with a needle, it is not going to help to keep asking them if it is hurting and freaking out, as this can then freak out the child. I understand they want to protect their child, but at some point they need to realize that we also want to protect their child. If parents keep asking them if it hurts, it really can make the child think "Wow, my dad thinks I'm in pain, maybe I am!".

One very helpful dad of a three-year-old started telling the boy a story right when I started the procedure. The child had only topical medicine but upon testing seemed to have no pain. I started suturing. The dad told a long story, a fantasy story that he was clearly making up on the spot, about a boy who was an adventurer. It had to do with a long journey, a castle, his fellow adventurers, treasure, etc. It was a long procedure but the story kept the boy mesmerized during the entire procedure. I actually found myself following the story and anxious to hear how it ended! What a fantastic dad this kid had.

Another mom stands out for the same reason. Her 13-year-old came in with a huge leg laceration that he had sustained while climbing on a fence. I was actually quite surprised by the size of it when the tech removed the dressing. On top of it, the boy seemed to be a high-stress type of kid, and was very nervous and tearful. Sometimes boys this age have an incredible fear of needles and procedures on their bodies. Teenage boys are well-known for actually fainting when we do procedures as any veteran nurse will tell you.

This boy's mother, when we started the procedure, started talking about family vacations they had taken, going through the trips step by step, and asking the boy if he remembered various parts of the trip. They had recently taken a trip through Canada with many family members, and she talked about funny things that had happened. I often talk as well during the procedure, but it was a very complex and deep laceration, and it really helped that I could concentrate completely on the laceration. I told her when we were done what a huge difference she had made for her kid. Because of her, he made it through a difficult procedure with no problem. Parents really are their child's best advocate in the Emergency Department.

Decisions

People often ask why I went into Emergency Medicine. When I made my decision, 25 years ago, there were several reasons.

I had started my clinical rotations in medical school, and the first one was internal medicine. I had a great chief resident, I've actually never met anyone like her before or since. She was tall, probably 5'11", blond, very outgoing, and never had anything negative to say. She always had a smile on her face and was best friends with everyone, from the Chief of Staff to the janitors. She started every day with a cup of water with three hot chocolate packages mixed into it, making hot chocolate the consistency of a thick soup.

She was going to go into Oncology. I can't imagine anyone better to take care of cancer patients. She was always well-read on all the literature, was a great teacher, and a genuinely compassionate person. All of the patients loved her. She seemed to love teaching us, and could break down the most complicated disease processes into basic forms for us, and had all sorts of helpful ways for us to remember the details. She was big on learning disease processes through pneumonics, which I don't usually like as a rule, but to this day I can faithfully recite the causes of Torsade de Pointes because of her, among other things. Truly amazing person.
Torsade De Pointes:

Phenothiazines
Other medications (tricyclic antidepressants)
Intracranial bleed
No known cause (idiopathic)
Type I anti-arrhythmics (quinidine, procainamide, dispyramide)
Electrolyte abnormalities
Syndrome of Prolonged QT (aka Long QT Syndrome)

Next, I did my surgery rotation. To my surprise I didn't love the operating room. I thought I would love it, but found it incredibly monotonous. Doing 12 gallbladder surgeries a day was mind-numbing, and there was almost zero interaction with awake patients. I really liked the surgeons though and felt that my thought processes were similar to theirs. I liked their pragmatic and straightforward approach to problems. Less thinking things out than Internal Medicine; the differential diagnoses list dropped to a few items that were most likely, and things were straightforward.

Next I did OB-GYN, and I thought this might be it for me. I started in a lovely community hospital where everyone was happy. All of the deliveries went off without a hitch and the most excitement was when someone had to get a c-section for failure to progress or a dad fainted during a delivery. The nurses were wonderful, and the docs were genuine, caring people. I loved the procedural part; setting up for a delivery, the step-by-step approach to the delivery, determining if there was a cord around the neck and gently reducing it, and suctioning and assessing the baby. I was in heaven.

For the second part of my rotation I went to our large inner city OB department. What I learned there (this was the 80's) is that cocaine is bad during pregnancy. Really bad. I think 75% of our patients had cocaine in their systems, and many of them would have abrupted (torn) their placentas.

One women who was five months pregnant was given 2 grams of cocaine (if I remember the amount correctly) by her boyfriend for her birthday and abrupted her placenta, killing both of her twins. We had women who had been pregnant 5, 6, 7 times and never delivered a live child secondary to a variety of factors. We had Social Workers reviewing every chart, CSD coming to the floor, and police in the room during some deliveries to take the baby away as soon as it was born, as there were court orders that the mom couldn't be around any children secondary to past abuse cases. I saw a mom get up immediately after her delivery to try and grab her baby and run.

It was a complete wake-up experience about a side of life I had never seen. On top of it, we had many patients who were just downright sick. Diabetes, renal failure, heart disease, plus most of them had social problems as well. Despite all this, I really liked the docs at this hospital and felt that I had definitely learned more than I had during the first, gentler portion of the rotation.

My next rotation was ICU. Loved it, the procedures, really sick patients, great attendings. The slightest difference in pulse or blood pressure and changes must be made immediately in medications or workup. The down side was the majority of our patients were extremely elderly and end-stage, and these were the days before advance directives and patient and family involvement in end-of-life decisions. We kept everyone alive whether they or their families wanted it or not. More on this later.

Next came trauma surgery. Now this was what I thought surgery would be like—meet the patient first time in the Emergency Department, make rapid assessments, rush to the OR without a firm diagnosis (again, these were the days before readily available CT—this is making me sound old), and very critical patients. Although I loved the OR my main job was helping take care of patients on the wards after surgery, and they were often quite sick. I really enjoyed that part and the surgeons were relieved that I could take care of the ward patients, as they didn't enjoy that part of their jobs as much as spending time in the OR.

My final rotation was Emergency Medicine. This was in a big, urban Emergency Department. The acuity of the average patient was not as high as trauma surgery, but there was a great mix of patients that I loved. Myocardial infarction at 6 am, then at 6:30 they were wheeled off and you would see a 3-year-old with an ear infection, then a 63-year-old patient with abdominal pain who you would diagnose with gallstones, then a teenage overdose. The range of patients, diagnoses, treatments, procedures, all mixed in with the typical Emergency Department drama, cemented my decision. In addition, I felt that it would be a better lifestyle for women at that time. We had already started a family and the "on or off" nature of Emergency Medicine seemed great to me. I did notice that there were almost no women in it at the time, which I still don't understand.

I felt like my mind opened up in the Emergency Department. I learned how to put symptoms with a diagnosis. Someone came in with leg pain, no trauma, swelling: Get an ultrasound, they may have a deep venous thrombosis. Someone came in with chest pain, EKG is normal but their pulse ox is 91% and they are on birth control: Get a VQ scan to rule out pulmonary embolus (we did more VQ scans then, now we do CTs usually). A patient came in confused, on multiple medications: Call the family, look for suicide notes, ask the police to go to the scene to look for pill bottles. The diagnostic and detective work was fascinating for me.

I also liked that you didn't have to check for insurance, you just treated everyone, and I enjoyed working with all socioeconomic levels. You might have a trauma patient who was in a motor vehicle accident in a Mercedes who came in wearing the most expensive clothes, and a patient in the next room who was a long-term alcoholic there for a head injury. It didn't matter, everyone was treated the same, and I loved that.

When I made my decision, the head of the OB department and the head of the surgery department both talked to me, basically stating that I was making a huge mistake. The OB doctor made the point that I would never have follow-up with my patients (largely true), and the surgeon made the point that I would only be temporizing medical conditions, rarely fixing them (largely true). But now, years later, I still feel it was the right decision for me.

Street People

Most of us perform our residency training at large, urban hospitals, and this was my experience. Because of that, we see a higher proportion of uninsured and homeless individuals than in most community hospitals. More alcoholism and drug abuse are encountered, and the patients who partake in that lifestyle are at higher risk of basically, everything medical or traumatic that can happen. Abscesses, head injuries, rape, broken bones, infections, assaults; this is the unfortunate result of the lifestyle these patients lead. Despite this many of these patients we see for years and years as they somehow manage to live day to day under difficult circumstances.

One patient we saw on an almost daily basis in our Emergency Department during residency was Henry, an elderly gentleman. He and his wife lived downtown, and were both chronic alcoholics. They were both homeless but occasionally found places to stay. They both had shopping carts they pushed around town.

Henry would come in almost daily because some good citizen would see him lying down on a street, possibly with vomit around him, and unconscious. Sometimes he would be seizing, because he had alcohol withdrawal seizures. The citizen would call 911, and then we would see Henry again, give him some IV Ativan for the seizures and a "banana bag" (an IV with various vitamins and minerals in it that benefits chronic alcoholics) and let him wake up. Sometimes he would need to be admitted, sometimes he would refuse and would leave, but always pleasantly. We would offer shelter placement but Henry and his wife, Marg, would both refuse as they didn't like the shelters.

Both he and his wife were very pleasant. They were always happy, and grateful to be cared for. This was in stark difference to most patients we saw in their situation.

One time I remember Marg, his wife, came in. I was quite new to the program, and didn't know her well yet. My fellow resident was caring for her. He complained as he told our attending (head physician) about her. "She is cussing at me, and tried to hit me. She scratched the nurse and needs to be restrained". Our wise attending, who had worked there 20 years, said immediately, "Oh, that can't be Marg. She is always sweet as can be. She must have something really wrong with her".

I saw the look of disgust on my fellow resident's face. This clearly was not scientific, or good medical practice, and it was obvious he didn't agree. "She is usually sweet, now she isn't, so there must be something wrong with her?" They went together to examine the patient. Sure enough, Marg was nasty to our attending, and tried to grab her arm. She was screaming and swinging at staff. Against the resident's protests, our attending ordered a stat brain CT, which showed a large subdural hemorrhage (a bleed on the brain). Marg must have fallen and hit her head. She was admitted and had neurosurgery, then was discharged in just a few days, completely back to her normal sweet self.

I had a one week vacation my 1st year of residence, which I was very thankful for as I was 6 weeks pregnant with my second child and suffering from horrible morning sickness. I spent the week resting and peacefully watching Sesame Street and playing with my three year old. My morning sickness I found to be much better when I wasn't running around at work with the smells at the hospital. However, the week was up, and I returned to the Emergency Department for a 7 am shift.

My first patient was coming by ambulance immediately, Code 3 (acute emergency, lights and sirens on). We heard the radio report that it was a patient whose leg had been severely traumatized. The patient was sleeping in a dumpster, and when the large garbage truck arrived that lifts the dumpster and dumps it into the trash compartment for compaction, they realized too late that there was a man in it. They heard screaming and stopped the compactor, but not before it had done significant damage.

Upon the paramedic's arrival, I was shocked to see it was Henry. The smell of the trash compactor, where he had been sleeping, immediately filled the Emergency Department and I felt my nausea rise. As the nurse started the IV's, and I ordered tests, morphine, and began examining him, I reached over and vomited in the trash can near the bed. I continued my exam as the surgeons arrived, and they took him immediately to the OR, to work on his severely mangled leg. It was a sad day for all of us.

After Henry was wheeled off to the OR, I went into the bathroom and vomited again. The trash compactor smell of rotting food was too much for me. I finished my shift, and found out in the middle of the day that they had to amputate Henry's leg above the knee. We all wondered what would happen to Henry now. Life is hard enough on the streets without having your leg amputated.

Henry recovered amazing well. He continued to frequent our Emergency Department on a routine basis. He would never consent to alcohol treatment, and I always thought both he and his wife's lives would be short-lived because of their lifestyle. He now had an artificial limb that he would frequently not wear, and would have sticking up out of his grocery cart and would use the grocery cart like a walker. Sometimes he lost the artificial leg and would come in without it, but he always somehow got it back.

About five years later, I was eating at a restaurant downtown with a friend. As we left the restaurant, I saw a dark shape approaching, limping, and pushing a shopping cart. I stopped talking and looked closely. It was Henry! I could not believe it. I approached him, and told him who I was. He acted like he remembered me though I wasn't sure. I asked about Marg, he assured me she was fine, just not with him tonight. He actually looked the same, and was his smiling and cheerful self.

Years later, I heard about a group of residents, I forget where, who celebrated the end of their residency with a party. They invited some of the "regulars", patients who sounded like Henry and Marg, to the party. This somehow made the news, and was viewed to be very inappropriate, apparently because it was felt to be demeaning to the patients. I felt some sympathy for the residents, assuming they did it for the reasons which I would like to believe. I learned so much from patients like this, and I really did feel they were a significant part of my education, especially as far as me learning that not everyone had the same lifestyle as me, nor wanted it, and that you can't always change that. You have to do whatever you can to help them and can't be judgmental of them though this can be very difficult. They do become part of your life and part of the Emergency Department that you will always remember.

One of the nurses in our department makes blankets every year for homeless patients. She sews pockets in the inside of the blankets for the alcohol bottles of the alcoholic patients. She makes the blankets then hands them out for free, including driving downtown and giving them to street people she sees. While many people would view that as enabling, the fact is that we often can't change what patients are going to do, even though we try. She just wants to take care of them.

Adrenaline

If you asked most Emergency Physician's, acute resuscitations are the part of the job that we most enjoy. To take an acutely ill patient, who is in acute respiratory failure or having an acute cardiac event, and to stabilize them with an emergency airway or with medications is challenging and fulfilling, and gives you a rush that is indescribable.

My favorite resuscitation ever, came on what had started as a fairly calm day in the Emergency Department. We were sitting (a rare event) at the nurse's station. I was looking up labs on patients I was caring for, and the nurse's were charting. Suddenly, a triage nurse burst through our double doors carrying a limp child, approximately two. Dad was behind her.

"He's in respiratory distress!" she said, obviously very concerned. We immediately placed him on the gurney, and began assessing him as we began to treat him. I opened his jaw, a nurse placed him on a monitor, and two nurses went to work on IV placement. He had a markedly slow respiratory rate, and had poor color. We immediately began "bagging" him, with a facemask and a hand-held bag that forces oxygen into his lungs, called an Ambu bag. The nurses rapidly got two IV's. I attempted to communicate with dad what we were doing, in brief updates.

Dad stood quietly, obviously distressed, and would nod his head as I would speak to him but didn't take his eyes off the child. We had to intubate the child (place a tube into his lungs) as his respiratory rate was not improving though his oxygen saturation had improved. We performed a rapid sequence intubation, which is where we give sedating and paralyzing medications in a rapid fashion, then intubate the child to breathe for him. This went smoothly and he was hooked up to a ventilator as we got a stat x-ray and blood work.

As the child stabilized, I could now ask the dad questions. Dad related to me now that the child had had a cold for several days. His only history was that he had been a "NICU" baby, on a ventilator for premature birth, but had not had any problems since then. His wife had stayed home from work yesterday with him and dad stayed home today. His respiratory effort had seemed to increase today so dad called his pediatrician, and was on the way to the pediatrician when he noticed the child seemed to be in acute distress, and came to the Emergency Department immediately instead of driving to the office, thankfully.

The child was admitted, diagnosed with RSV (Respiratory Syncytial Virus), kept on a ventilator for several days and then went home. The staff received a lovely letter from mom, showing dad on the couch snuggling a sleeping, peaceful child. "I assume that the reason you went into medicine is to deal with this type of emergency. I want to thank you for your decision, and for your skills and training. Every minute when we look at our child, we realize what our lives would have been like without him, and we feel blessed." It was a moving and touching letter and I still keep it in my mailbox at work.

There is now a fairly new immunization against RSV, which is very helpful in children who were NICU babies or kiddos with chronic lung problems. RSV is a disease which has always really scared me because kids can change so fast with it. When older kids get RSV it is usually just a "cold", and nothing to worry about. When premature babies or kids with other medical problems get it, they can look like they just have a cold, but can then have "apneic episodes", where they can stop breathing. These are unexpected and unpredictable.

A less fortunate resuscitation that took quite an ugly turn I also remember. We learned from the radio that we were expecting an ambulance, Code 3, with a 3-year-old with respiratory distress. On their arrival, the paramedics were bagging the patient to assist his breathing. The child was limp. They said the parents were driving on the highway, but had pulled over when they noticed the child was having trouble breathing and called 911.

We immediately placed the child on our heart monitor the second the paramedics arrived, assisting with the child's airway by continuing bagging with an Ambu bag, and placing an IV. Mom and dad arrived in the room. They began screaming at our staff and grabbing at the child. I have always prided myself on not ever asking a family to leave the room, and I communicated with them to explain what we were doing, thinking it would calm them down. They continued screaming and pushing. On top of it all, I was having troubles with the child's airway. We could always bag him and were careful to keep his oxygen levels up between intubation attempts, but I was on my second attempt at intubation. We had to frequently suction him as he was vomiting. The dad became increasingly agitated, and threw himself on the floor. He screamed that he was going to sue me. He then called someone on his cell phone and was screaming into the phone.

As the family continued screaming and grabbing at the child, I was able to intubate on my third attempt. It was complicated because the child had vomit in his mouth and the vomit would accumulate as fast as I could suction it out. Finally though the tube was in proper position.

As we stabilized the child, I made plans to admit him and attempted to talk with the family. They were still agitated and still screaming at us. I told the pediatric attending about the situation.

The attending physician called me two days later. In a bizarre turn of events, it turned out the family had given the child a type of toxin (a poison) and had admitted doing it when confronted with the laboratory proof. Police had been contacted and the attending physician wanted to know if I could relate the events of the resuscitation to the police.

I did speak to them, though I never heard what finally happened with this family. It was the only time I should have asked a family to leave or had them removed from the Emergency Department as they actually disrupted the resuscitation. Thank God everything went well for that child, and at least he had a medical recovery.

Overall though, I'm a big believer of having the closest family members in the room during resuscitation. When I was a resident that was never done. The family always had to wait in the waiting room. The first time I had a mom in the room was when the mom had refused to leave the child when the paramedics arrived, and stayed in the ambulance with her child. The paramedics quickly let us know that when they arrived. I made a rapid decision to let her stay in the room. Fortunately there was a great nurse who explained things to the mom as we went, as some of it can appear very disturbing to family members, such as putting down an endotracheal tube into their loved ones mouth, or performing a lumbar puncture (spinal tap). But the mom did great, and I knew it was because of the nurse's explanations.

There is a concern that a family will misunderstand or overreact to something going on, and I have seen that happen, but it is very rare. I had a 17-year-old come in with meningococcus, a deadly bacterial infection that often affects teens. We had no heads up that they were coming in as they came by private auto, and during the initial scramble the nurse tripped over a monitor line that had just been placed, pulling it off. No big deal at all, that kind of stuff happens, but the dad freaked out about it. We rapidly calmed him down, and I told him this was the best nurse in the hospital which was true. The kid did great thank God, but you can see where an emotionally overwrought parent could take one little event like that and think that it caused a problem if their child didn't do well.

I personally think if it was my family member though, I would want to know how hard everyone was working, how many people were in the room, and I would want to see the looks on their faces. I definitely can't see myself waiting outside in a waiting room.

Also, sometimes family members will tell us very important information during the resuscitation. Last year I was resuscitating a 45-year-old man who arrested at home. I knew he had leukemia and had been getting chemotherapy for that, and had even undergone a stem-cell transplant, but didn't know anything else in his history. I only knew he had collapsed at home.

His wife arrived five minutes after the patient, and we couldn't get any heart activity back at all on this guy. I had her brought back into the room, and she told me that he had been very weak and fatigued from his treatment, and had been in bed for days, barely getting out. Today he complained of leg cramps in one leg, then had onset of right posterior back pain that came on all of a sudden. She tried rubbing his back to help, then he had cardiac arrest.

Everything suddenly became clear. He had thrown a huge pulmonary embolus (blood clot). Being bedridden and having cancer are two major risk factors. Blood clots form in your legs, that is why he had the cramping. He had then thrown the clot up to his chest, the back part of his chest, which he interpreted as back pain. We continued to try to resuscitate him without success for over half an hour, but could get nothing back at all.

I explained to the wife that this was probably a blood clot, and this gave her some understanding of what had happened. We explained that there was nothing else she could have done, as it had clearly been a massive clot, so hopefully this gave her some small element of understanding of what had happened to her husband. In addition, she didn't want an autopsy, and I felt comfortable that now we knew a cause of death.

Having family members in the room is one of the biggest changes I've experienced in my career, and it has definitely been one of the best changes in my opinion.

One thing that none of us like in the Emergency Department is when a patient that we are caring, who comes in alert, takes a turn for the worse. Fortunately it is a rare event, but none of us like having a patient who comes in looking OK then has something happen, as you always feel like you should have been able to predict it.

I took care of a 2 month old boy, brought in by his mother for "abdominal pain". I spent a lot of time talking with the mom about why she thought he was having abdominal pain, and she had difficulty describing it, but generally it sounded like he had been fussy and maybe colicky. He had a cold for several days. I ordered blood work, a urine test, an acute abdomen series x-ray (includes a chest and abdomen) and an ultrasound of his abdomen. He looked great, had a little runny nose, but no fever and stable vital signs. His blood work was normal. His ultrasound was normal. I thought his x-ray had a little too much gas in his bowel, more than usual. Mom still felt he was having pain, so I asked Dr. Elver, our pediatric surgeon to see him.

I called Dr. Elver at about two in the morning and fortunately she was upstairs in the hospital seeing another patient. Dr. Elver came down, spent a long time with the patient, examined the baby, and reviewed all of the tests. She felt we could safely discharge the patient and was going to see the baby the next day in her office to recheck him. She couldn't find any abdominal pain on her examination, agreed that the baby looked great, and all of his tests were normal.

I talked with mom again who felt comfortable with this plan. In the meantime though the nurse was very busy and could not get in to do the discharge with the associated paperwork right away. I was feeling bad that the discharge was taking so long; it was so late and they had been there for so long. But it is important that the patient and family wait to get all the information they need and get their vital signs re-taken before they go.

"We need you in room 15 right away!" a nurse yelled at me. I ran to the room, and realized on the way there it was the baby. When I walked in, he was blue, and the nurse was positioning him for resuscitation. As we started Ambu bagging his ventilations, I asked what happened. "He just stopped breathing and turned blue when I was holding him on my lap!" the mom said. Dr. Elver had rushed into the room as she had been doing paperwork and assisted us. She looked as shocked as I felt.

Within just a few puffs from the Ambu bag, the child began breathing on his own. He perked up and looked the same as he had before. His vital signs were stable; but my blood pressure was about 250/150. We admitted him to the Intensive Care Unit, where he also was diagnosed with RSV. Ultimately, it all came down to just that, the RSV. The abdominal pain never came to anything. The baby did fine and went home.

I did feel the baby had guardian angels, first his mom, who I think just knew something was wrong; and second, a real guardian angel who kept the nurse from coming in the room right away to discharge him. That extra half an hour let him have his respiratory arrest in the Emergency Department and not in the car on their way home. Dr. Elver and I had our own little debriefing session, but in this case all it came down to was being lucky. We both felt that the symptoms the child had come in with were very atypical and that we could not have expected what had happened.

It was about 4 in the morning when this happened, usually the time I need to start drinking coffee and get a little caffeine in me to finish up the last hours of my night shift. That morning I definitely did not need the coffee and it took about two extra hours to wind down to get to sleep that morning. Four in the morning is not the right time to get a big adrenaline rush.

Hospice

The other situation which comes up almost every day with resuscitations is an elderly patient presenting in acute respiratory failure or cardiac failure. Usually they come by ambulance and we don't know their "DNR" (Do Not Resuscitate) status; sometimes it is on our computer but often it is not. There is an effort going on to make it centralized information, on a state computer website, but this is in the early stages. Some patients have not been at a hospital before so this information has never been entered, or they keep the papers at home in a drawer or safe deposit box, and the paramedics have no way of knowing where to find the information. If no family arrives to tell us of an advanced directive, of course we must resuscitate this patient.

When I was in medical school over 20 years ago, we resuscitated everyone, no matter what they or their families wanted, and even if they had a terminal condition. Our society has now had increasing awareness of this, and patients fill out advanced directives stating what they want. They can specify if they want everything done, or if they don't want heroic measures such as CPR (chest compressions and medications to re-start their heart) or to be on a ventilator. They can even make the care very specific such as they would want antibiotics and full treatment but not be on long-term life support, or not want tube feedings.

Several years ago, I had an elderly, frail woman, about 95-years-old, present in marked respiratory distress. The patient had an extensive history of severe congestive heart failure ever since she had a large heart attack several years ago. She was now in florid congestive heart failure with fluid filling her lungs. You could hear it throughout her lungs when listening with a stethoscope.

The paramedics had started her on Lasix in the ambulance, and we gave her more quickly through her IV and ordered a stat portable chest x-ray that would be done in the room so we didn't have to move her. The paramedics didn't know her DNR status. They said the daughter lived next door to the patient and would be right in. "Great", I thought to myself. I would have to make a decision in the next few minutes on whether she was responding to the medication or would need intubation, and often there is an amazing delay in getting family members there. However, this daughter arrived within minutes. At this point I explained the patient needed immediate intubation, as she wasn't responding to the medication, and she would need to be put on a ventilator, which is of course, life support.

I spoke with the daughter. "Oh, she wouldn't want that. Dad died several months ago, and she wants to join him," she explained. I asked if she had DNR paperwork and the daughter assured me she did but she had no idea where it was. She knew her mom was DNR though. I asked if I should discuss it with other family, but she was the only child and felt comfortable with the decision. These are decisions we have to make every day, but I usually trust the family and have never had a problem thank God. If there is any hesitation, or they want to talk to Uncle Jim or a cousin in Florida first before a decision is made, I always go full-court press on resuscitation until everyone is on the same page.

I spoke with the patient then. On high-flow oxygen, she looked slightly improved, but was still gasping when she tried to speak. I asked her if she would want us to put her on life support, to help her breathing. She grabbed both my hands. "Sweetie, please don't do that. I just want to go. I want to see my husband. Please don't do that." The daughter agreed. We talked about the fact that none of us wanted the patient to be in any distress, which she was in now. We agreed to start her on a Morphine drip. When someone is in acute respiratory distress from congestive heart failure, morphine can make the "work" of breathing much less and makes the patient more comfortable, but the risk is that it can decrease respiratory drive. I explained the risk to both of them, and they accepted the risks and wanted to start the drip.

The morphine drip helped this patient tremendously. When I walked by later, she was holding hands with her daughter and looking at her, and breathing much more comfortably.

Some families and patients want to go full court press no matter what. I had a 94-year-old Russian speaking patient come in several years ago, accompanied by her son. He had a very commanding presence is what I remember about him. His mother was tiny, frail, and had very severe abdominal pain. Evaluation revealed very abnormal electrolytes on her blood work, and a CT scan that showed very severe pancreatitis, with edema (swelling) all around the pancreas and changes in her fat around it. In addition her blood work revealed probable infection. Although I didn't feel she would be in imminent danger, I wanted to convey to the son how sick she was, and in a 94-year-old frail woman this could be potentially fatal. Since she was being admitted to the ICU, I asked if she had an advanced directive that I should place on the chart. He asked what that was and I explained it; that some patients wouldn't want chest compressions or to be on life support if they took a major turn for the worse, and that we would abide by that.

"Wouldn't that be called murder?" He asked. His question actually left me speechless for a minute, a rare event. When I could discuss it with him further, he felt that anything short of everything we could in modern medicine would not be acceptable. People just have different opinions on these things. The important thing is discussing them ahead of time with the patient and family to be sure you do what the patient would want. You don't want to be in a situation in the hospital where you go against the wishes of the patient and their families if an emergency happens.

The important thing for patients is to discuss it with your family members ahead of time. If a 90-year-grandpa has had metastatic cancer for four years, has failed every type of surgery, radiation therapy, and chemotherapy, then at some point his end-of-life wishes should be discussed with him by his own doctor and his family. If he wants everything done including the ventilator and chest compressions, that is his choice, but often people's wishes in this case are to be comfortable and be with family, and of course to have no pain. It is always just a bit surprising to me in this type of situation if there has never been a discussion at all, and no one thought grandpa was ever going to really go, ever. That then puts everyone in the position of having to decide what grandpa would want if there is an emergency, and if it isn't clear, we have to go full-court press.

I recently had a 35-year-old male in full cardiac arrest arrive at 9 pm at night. The paramedics said he was vomiting blood and had esophageal cancer. He was also severely developmentally delayed. One of the staff wondered aloud why there was no DNR paperwork on him. When the paramedics arrived, the patient obviously had congenital abnormalities, weighed about 90 pounds and was completely jaundiced. He had lost his pulse and had no spontaneous respirations. When I listened to his chest with my stethoscope, I noticed that I could see every rib. The paramedics said the patient's brother wanted him to be a full code. We therefore continued the code. Despite chest compressions, ventilation, and ACLS medications, we could not get any consistent heart activity back. I left my partner to run the code while I went to talk with the brother.

When I met the brother, he was pacing in the family room, a small waiting area for family members. I took his hands and we talked about what had happened tonight at home. He told me that his brother was severely developmentally delayed and functioned at the level of a three year old. Their parents had died a few years prior and he had taken care of "Marky" since that time. Then Marky had gotten esophageal cancer and had failed multiple chemotherapy agents. I updated him on the resuscitation efforts, and he immediately wanted to come back to the room. He understood that further resuscitation was futile, and he wanted to see his brother.

We went back to the room, and he took the patient's head gently in his hands. "I love you so much Marky. Mommy and daddy love you too. You are going to go to heaven with Mommy and Daddy and all your uncles and aunts. Everyone wants you in heaven. It's OK to go. I love you so much. You've been the best thing that has ever happened to me." He then signaled for me to stop resuscitation efforts which we did.

There was no one in the room without tears at this point. This case proved to me that doing whatever the family wants is the right thing. I personally would not have chosen to do aggressive resuscitation on a terminal cancer patient who had failed all prior treatments, but this brother did, and it gave him a chance to tell his brother goodbye. It also showed all of us a glimpse of what it is all really about, the love of one family member for another that is completely unconditional.

The whole process of dealing with death issues and family members in the Emergency Department takes much longer than simply resuscitating a patient. I know that sounds callous, but in a rushed shift where you have 15 other patients and 30 in the waiting room, this does cross your mind. But sometimes I think I have done a bigger service letting patients and their families have a comfortable, pain free death when they have a terminal, irreversible condition, than in prolonging the inevitable with our ventilators and resuscitation medications, if that is what they and their families want. Spending time with a family member when the inevitable happens and letting them spend time with a family member is irreplaceable. I really take pride in doing everything we can to make these patients as comfortable as we can and giving them all the support they need in their final hours. A quiet room, your pastor with you, holding hands with your family, and having no pain. There are worse ways to go. This has been a big change for most practitioners that are my age, and something that really didn't happen 20 years ago. It is a big improvement for patients and families in controlling their own care and their end-of-life quality.

Coping Mechanisms

Staff who work in the Emergency Department often use a variety of coping mechanisms to deal with the situations we see there.

Humor is probably the most common coping mechanism that I see. We all do it to a certain degree; but it has to be done absolutely out of patient ear-shot and there is a fine line between being collegial and being inappropriate, though I will admit that line is very often crossed and I can't lie about that.

One young woman I took care of stated she felt like she had something in her vagina. She had no idea what it was, but it felt like a pressure.

I wondered if she had an abscess or a prolapsed bladder, but when I inserted the speculum, I saw a white object with the words "Top Flite" on it. After some difficulty, I was able to remove the glistening white golf ball from her vagina. I didn't ask her about how it got there and she didn't volunteer any information as I plopped it onto the tray next to me. I just talked to her for awhile, gave her warning signs about infection as she looked down at the floor, and told her she didn't have to wait for the nurse to discharge her in order to save her the embarrassment of having to talk to one more person. She gladly dressed and made her escape.

One of my male partners walked up to me as I was carrying the tray down the hallway. "What's that?" he asked. "A golfball, what do you think it is?" I said sarcastically. I told him a brief run down on the story. "How'd you get it out of there?" he wanted to know what gynecological instrument I had used.

"A Nine iron" I said and walked off.

I've had patients use humor too, which I really appreciate. One gentleman I took care of, a local TV news anchor, had a large laceration on the back of his head from a fall. When I tried to look, I couldn't see the laceration through his hair. Finally he told me, "Look doc, just between you and me, I wear a hair piece. We're going to have to get it unglued for you to see it, but the blood is dripping down so I know I've got a cut". He laughed and told me I could use the information to bribe him. He was a great sport about it.

What I fear about humor in the Emergency Department though, is that crossing of the line. We always have to remember that the patient has a right to privacy, and not to laugh at unfortunate situations. I even felt I crossed the line with the golf ball when I thought about it later.

The first time I was ever in a pediatric trauma, it was a 4-year-old, unconscious after being hit by a car while riding his trike. I was only a medical student. The thought of having a critical child in this situation was overwhelming but I tried my best to be completely professional. My job was to check the child's blood pressure and pulse. As I looked at the child, I thought, subconsciously, oh, he has long dirty nails. He must not be well cared for and this is why this happened. In years to come, I would realize that is how I rationalized that something like this could happen. Even as I thought it I felt guilty for thinking it because I knew it was wrong. I had to get through this situation without thinking that this could be my child, and that is how my subconscious took over.

I think now that it sounds awful that I had those thoughts, but it got me through the code and what I needed to do. After the first few pediatric traumas and codes, I could handle them in a professional manner, and though I am always having deep emotions about any resuscitation especially pediatrics, I can now usually, though not always, segregate them in a different part of my brain so that I can handle the situation. I think that is what we all do. After about 10 years of practice I could run a pediatric resuscitation without later going to the bathroom by myself for a minute to get myself back together, then back to work.

To this day, though, there are the occasional cases that I can't completely process, and I know other doctors and nurses who feel the same way.

I had a two month old child come in this year, who had been found not breathing at home. The paramedics were breathing for her with a bag and mask, and performing chest compressions upon arrival. After I intubated her and got a good IO line (an IV that goes in the leg bone), we got a pulse and a blood pressure back. Although we were temporarily relieved, a brain CT that we got a few minutes later showed a huge skull fracture and a very large bleed into her brain that we knew would prove fatal. Child abuse from a babysitter. If she lived she would never walk or talk. We silently continued the resuscitation efforts and she was transferred to the pediatric ICU where she was later declared brain dead and taken off life support.

After she had gone upstairs, the charge nurse planned a "debriefing" where we all go talk about the case. The two nurses and tech, who have worked there 40 years among the three of them, and me, all looked at each other then glanced away without talking. We had just spent time with the mom (who was not the abuser, she had just returned to work after maternity leave), and had just finished this futile resuscitation. None of us could go to a debriefing, none of us could talk about it. We said we would go the next week but we never did. Although we should probably all have gone, there are some things that are too painful, too terminal, too sad for words. And in those situations there are no coping mechanisms that are going to help you feel any differently. As I write this now, a year later, I still feel a horrible feeling welling up for this child and for her family. I just can't process it completely and maybe never will.

Recently, I had a child rushed to the Emergency Department from upstairs in the hospital where he was receiving a CT scan of his head. His pediatrician had ordered it but he had started seizing in the CT. He came down with no IV in, actively seizing and turning blue.

We resuscitated him and gave him Ativan and Fosphenytoin to stop his seizing. The resuscitation went perfectly smoothly, amazingly smoothly. Usually there is some stressful event for us practitioners such as the IO isn't working right, it is a difficult intubation, or you can't get blood drawn, but everything went like clockwork. We were all feeling that exhilaration that you get from a successful resuscitation.

I then asked for someone to get me the CT report from the scan he was having upstairs. Our secretary came in the room and handed me the phone with the radiologist on it. "Mary, he's got a mass, and it looks like it may have bled into it. Actually, it looks like it may even be two tumors that are joined". I felt my stomach sinking as he talked.

I went out of the room to talk to the parents. I had met them during the resuscitation, and though I always let parents stay in the room somehow they were now standing at the doorway, slightly outside of the room, probably because there were 10-15 people in the room working on the child. They had probably been trying to stay out of the way. I told them the details of the resuscitation, and I told them there was an abnormal CT scan.

I looked at the mom and then the dad in the eyes, and I told them their child had what looked like a brain mass with possible bleeding. The dad had tears in his eyes; the mom just looked shocked. I told them we wouldn't know if it was malignant or not until we did more tests. I talked for a few minutes about what we would be doing, the admission, the ICU, etc, and asked if they had questions.

"No,", the mom said, "thank you so much for everything. Thank you so much for explaining everything to us", she said very formally and politely, almost robotically. Then she said, "Well, I do have a question…" "What is it?" I asked.

Her voice started, cracked, then sobs poured out of her. "Why did this happen? Why did this happen? Why did this happen?" She asked this over and over, as her body bent over involuntarily and she wrapped her arms around herself. This really got to all of us in the room, because she had been trying to hold it together so hard, then she just completely broke down.

I told her that was absolutely no reason that this happened. And that was the truth. Sometimes things happen and we don't know why, and there is nothing anyone has done wrong, there is just no reason. As patients and doctors, we always want to know why something bad happened, and sometimes there is something we've done wrong, or something that happened to us, but for most disease processes, it just happens for absolutely no reason that we can think of. Why did this child have this happen and other children don't? There is no reason.

I went home and the interaction kept popping into my head, as I thought about the family. The next day I called and talked to the neurosurgeon who confirmed in his opinion that it was a brain tumor and they were taking the child to surgery shortly.

Sometime later, several weeks I believe, I showed up for work and looked at my mail. A discharge summary had come on the child. It wasn't a tumor, it was a bizarre infected area with an abscess from presumed bacterial seeding. The child had gotten a bacterial infection, the bacteria migrated to the arteries of the brain, and had formed an area of infection. It had gotten big enough that it had bled into the area. The area was resected and the child went home without neurological deficits, completely normal. It was a very rare situation and I had never seen anything like it in my practice.

I was elated, almost giddy. I had been feeling so horrible. I let the nurses know who were involved, and started my day.

My first patient after I left my office was a 28-year-old asthmatic respiratory arrest patient, found down by his mother, who could not be resuscitated by paramedics and was in full cardiac arrest. Although we eventually got his heart started again I knew it would be futile, that he would be brain dead. He had been "down" in the field for over

20 minutes with no pulse, possibly longer. The he had CPR and ACLS medications with paramedics for about 30 minutes. Having that long of period with no good blood supply to the brain, plus whatever time he was on the floor of his bedroom with no one knowing, it is not going to end well. We started the "Rapid Cooling" protocol, which is a new thing we do to cool patient's body temperatures down to protect their brain, and in some cases does seem really helpful, but this was just a long time to have no pulse.

The swing in emotions is extreme in the Emergency Department. I was so elated, and then within 10 minutes had this situation with a distraught family, expressing to them that I did not think this would be OK for this patient. The fact is, you want to be honest with the patient's families, and they want to now what you think is the truth. Sometimes we are right and sometimes we are wrong in what we think will happen, but sometimes we do know, and it is not what anyone wants to hear. But you have to say it anyway.

The Strangest Case

People often ask me, what is the strangest case I've ever seen in the Emergency Department. Actually, to be specific, they ask what is the grossest thing. But the strangest case I've ever had is far more interesting and one that I think of often.

We had a report that an ambulance was coming with an unresponsive 32-year-old woman in respiratory distress. Asthma? I wondered. Pneumonia? Their report wasn't very enlightening. I resumed charting, and several minutes looked up to see a gurney being pushed into the acute resuscitation room, with an emaciated, bright orange patient.

"They didn't tell me it was a cancer patient", I thought to myself. I approached the paramedics and asked for report.

"She has brain cancer, and has been down in Mexico at a cancer clinic for the cure", the paramedic said, breathless. "She's been there for about a year and just got home. She's staying with her brother, he'll be right in. She started getting confused and sleepy today, and they called when they couldn't wake her up".

The nurse had her on a monitor and she already had an IV in from the paramedics. Her oxygen level on the pulse oximetry was only 82% despite the high flow oxygen. "She needs to be intubated, does the family want that?" I asked paramedics. My concern was that if she was a terminal cancer patient, she may have plans to not to receive "heroic" life-saving measures, such as life support. "They didn't talk about it, I don't know", the paramedic said. The patient's respiratory status looked very concerning to me, and appeared to be deteriorating. Her pupils responded sluggishly. I had our respiratory therapist start Ambu bagging her and setting up for intubation.

Fortunately, the family arrived right then, the brother and sister-in-law. They told me that two years ago, while living in another city, she had a malignant melanoma removed from her forearm. Several months later, she went in for a CT scan for a headache. They found a mass, and it was discussed with her that her malignant melanoma had spread. She was to have other testing, the start chemotherapy and have brain surgery immediately. Panicked, the patient went home and looked for other alternatives. She found a clinic in Mexico on-line, that offered "cures" for cancer. She flew down immediately, and never had surgery or chemo.

In Mexico, they had her "fast" for two weeks. Then she had daily carrot juice enemas and coffee enemas, combined with drinking larges amount of carrot juice and coffee to "cleanse her system". Her only other foods were vegetables. She had done this for almost a year, and that is why she appeared so skinny and orange now.

She had just returned home for the holidays yesterday. I asked the family if she would want to be intubated. They really didn't know. In Emergency Department language, that means "yes". If there is no plan or agreement when the patient comes in, no paperwork for DNR status, the patient will typically get intubated and put on life support.

I quickly intubated her, put her on a ventilator and ordered a stat CT scan. When I pulled up the images, I was shocked to see how large the tumor was. It was forcing her brain to "herniate", basically forcing her brain into the spinal cord area.

We gave her Decadron, a steroid, through her IV to decrease the swelling and I called our neurosurgeon. The neurosurgeon I called and I had a longstanding relationship, nearly all bad. I called him and related the situation. Unfortunately there was just no way to make this story not sound strange. He yelled, "I can't believe you 're calling me about a terminal cancer patient! What do you want me to do, operate on her and make her live three more days?" and hung up the phone on me.

I had our secretary call him back. I explained that the family wanted us to attempt treatment, could he just come in and look at the scan and talk to the family, as I felt the patient and family needed a neurosurgical consultation. "Click", the receiver went. I went back to check on the patient as I had our secretary place another call.

My friendly neurosurgeon called back. I picked up the phone and began my begging routine again. Click. Right then I needed to go check on another patient; fine, that would give me a minute to think about my next move.

Five minutes later, while I was in with the other patient, I saw Dr. Tal, my neurosurgeon walking in, dressed in his typical suit and tie. "Mary!" he said pleasantly. "I apologize so much. Please forgive me. Now where is this patient of yours?" Though this sounds crazy, this was typical for our interactions. Once he got there he would be very apologetic and pleasant, not the same guy as over the phone. I took him to look at the CT, in those days they were still on film copies, not on the computer. That makes me sound old.

He looked at it for 2 seconds. "That is not malignant melanoma. That is just a meningioma", he declared. I stared blankly at it, with my training I could not make the differentiation but he could easily. A meningioma is a benign condition, basically a non-cancerous tumor that either causes no problems, or rarely may cause headaches and the like so is removed, but it will not spread. This one had just grown much bigger than anything I had ever seen. If the patient had had the initial surgery as proposed, it would have been biopsied, found to be not malignant melanoma, and she would not have needed chemotherapy. This tumor was completely unrelated to her prior cancer diagnosis of malignant melanoma.

As it was though, it was huge, and pushing pressure on her brainstem. Dr. Tal talked with the family, and took her immediately to the OR.

Now, as I have complained bitterly about Dr. Tal, I must tell the rest of the story. Technically, he was the best neurosurgeon on the staff. If I had a brain tumor, I would go to him. His patients always did well. He just had gotten to the end of his career, and hated late night Emergency Department calls, which truth be told, were never straight-forward, often from uninsured patients, and often involved alcohol. He retired about five years after this case. While I don't miss the phone call interactions, he was a great neurosurgeon.

I thought about this lady often the next few days. I felt she would still do poorly, and I thought it was sad she had given up what may now be the last year of her life to spend in a clinic out of the country, away from her family.

Several shifts later, a nurse told me I had a visitor. I went out to the nursing station and saw a patient standing there smiling, with an orange tan. It dawned on me at that point that this was the patient. She told me she had the surgery and woke up the next day, and felt great. Her family had come down with her to meet us. We talked for awhile, and I told her what I had been thinking about, that I was so glad she hadn't spent that year for nothing in Mexico.

She looked at me blankly, then said, "Oh, no. That is what helped me. The treatments converted my cancer into non-cancer. All that year, when I was taking the treatments, they told me that would hap-pen, and now it has.". She was so happy, as was her family, that I just smiled and was happy with them. They walked out of the Emergency Department, back into their lives. All I could think of is, you can't argue with success.

The runner-up story for strangest case I have had also had to do with Dr. Tal. The daughter of one of our nurses came in. She was 24, and kept getting headaches when she used a "rowing machine", a type of exercise equipment that she had at home. Everytime she used it she got a headache. "Stop using it" seems like a logical answer, but as she seemed very concerned we went ahead and got a CT scan.

The patient didn't even need pain medication, as she didn't have a headache now. She went off to CT scan, and about an hour later the radiologist called me. "She has an arachnoid cyst, its pretty big", was his response.

I thought about this. Weird. We see these from time to time, and they are usually thought to be an "incidental finding", something that is just there since birth but doesn't really cause problems. It probably wasn't related to her headache at all. An arachnoid cyst is made from a layer of tissue that covers our brain, and is filled with fluid. Usually they are just no big deal. I thought about it more. Why was she having a headache now? Could it be that the rowing machine somehow was causing pressure to build up? Maybe I would just run it by the neuro-surgeon to arrange follow-up for her.

I called Dr. Tal. He pulled up the CT on his home computer. "Just put her in", he said. I was really surprised. "Really? I didn't think these were such a big deal usually..." I thought he would just tell me to send the patient home and that he would see her in the office, or I thought he would yell at me for calling about this, but I didn't expect him to want to admit her. "Just admit her." "Click", the phone went dead.

I went ahead and admitted her to Dr. Tal, and promptly forgot about her. At about 2 in the morning, I heard, "Code 99 overhead". This is when there is a cardiopulmonary arrest in the hospital and the Emergency Physician responds to these. I ran up the stairs and to the patient's room.

To my surprise and dismay, it was the young patient with the arachnoid cyst. She was clearly in respiratory failure. As the Respiratory Therapist set up my equipment for intubation, I glanced at her eyes. One of her pupils was blown. "Shit!" I thought, or maybe I said it out loud, I'm not sure.

I yelled for someone to call Dr. Tal at home, and intubated the patient. I ordered IV Decadron and Mannitol for her to decrease brain swelling.

Within about 2 minutes, Dr. Tal arrived in the room. "How did you get here so fast?" I asked him, shocked. "I need you to take her to the OR". I learned later he lived right up behind the hospital.

"I know, they are ready for us," he said calmly.

They immediately wheeled the patient off to the OR.
The next day I was working, and I went in early to check on her. I was really, really worried that she wouldn't have a neurologic recovery. I felt like shit as she was one of my nurse's daughters, and though I was at least glad I called the neurosurgeon for a consult, to have had this event happen was horrible.

When I arrived in the ICU, she was in the very first room on the right side of the hall. To my shock, she was sitting up, watching a TV show, and laughing, with her mother sitting in a chair in the room.

I went in and talked with them for a while, and was so relieved that I could not believe it. I still had more questions than answers. What had made Dr. Tal worry about this arachnoid cyst, when we see them all of the time and they are no problem? Why had the patient suddenly had respiratory arrest from it? I think the answer was that hers was unusually big, and it was indeed building up pressure that was exacerbated by the rowing machine. I still don't know the answers to this day, but I am thankful that Dr. Tal took the time to look at this on his computer at home when I didn't know the answer, that he was impressed by the size and position of it, and I am really glad that he lived so close to the hospital.

The grossest thing I ever saw is an easy one. I was taking care of a lady during residency. She came in with a long skirt. I had already read her chart and read that she had severe lymphedema, which is severe swelling, of her legs. She had a history of extensive travel, some type of missionary work. She was also diabetic. The nurse's note stated that she was worried her legs were infected.

I talked with her a while. I did notice a bit of a foul odor in the room. She said her legs were hurting and she had noticed redness. When I went to examine the skin on her legs, there were deep indentations in her lymphedema, kind of like cellulite but much deeper. I was looking at them closely when I saw movement. I thought I was mistaken and looked closer, and then I realized what she had. Myiasis. Maggots isn't the scientific word, but that is what she had.

I felt like I was losing my composure for a minute, mainly because I was worried about how I would describe to her what she had, and I didn't want her to be upset. I forced myself to pull it together and explain it to her, and she took it very well. I got a dermatology consult for her, the closest I ever got to ordering a stat dermatology consult, and as we were at a teaching hospital they were very interested and helpful for her. The patient also did have a severe infection of the skin on her legs and had to be admitted to the hospital. The dermatologist explained to her that this problem is very difficult to get rid of.

Whenever I have a patient with lice or scabies, or any type of skin infection, I find myself scratching for the rest of my shift. Others have told me they do the same thing. Even when I think of this poor lady now I start itching.

Chest pain and gratitude

On the last two hours of a busy shift, I picked up yet another chart. All of my patients had been very sick as I was on the "critical" side of the Emergency Department. The new chart said "chest pain", with a 53-year-old male. I went to see him. He was there with his wife. He was a large, almost 6'5", overweight gentleman, who had very slow speech and a mild speech impediment. .

He told me about his chest pain, then I began asking questions to understand the type of pain better. "Well, it started at work…" he started, and went on to slowly explain what it felt like.

With every question, he would patiently explain his symptoms to me with his slow calm speech. Anyone who knows me will tell you I am the most hyperactive person they have ever known, and I talk and move extremely fast. I had seven other sick patients out there, and in this room we were moving in slow motion. I could hear the chart printer clicking, printing out new charts as we talked.

I forced myself to sit quietly as he went over his symptoms, answered my questions on his past history and risk factors (he had high cholesterol and hypertension), and also had a smoking history (stopped two years ago). His dad had a stent at age 53, so he had a positive family history which always really worries me.

I told him his EKG done at triage was normal, but I wanted to check a troponin (an enzyme the heart releases into the blood stream if the heart is having anginal chest pain) and an x-ray. He thanked me and agreed. We gave him aspirin and ordered the blood work.

The blood work came back negative, but the way he described his symptoms really concerned me. He had felt like someone had a knee on his chest when he had the pain at work, where he worked as a welder. I told him that despite the negative blood work, and normal EKG, I felt we should admit him. It was 6 pm, I couldn't do a stress test because they closed at 5, so we would admit him for more blood work and a stress test the following day.

This is such a common occurrence that I felt like I was on autopilot as I explained it. Near the end, he unexpectedly grabbed my hand. He began having tears, as did his wife. "Thank you so much for listening to me", he said. "And thank you for caring about me and for all the tests you are doing".

I was somewhat taken aback, I hadn't really expected this as he had been very unemotional up to this point. I thanked him for saying that, and we talked about what would happen in the hospital, and that I would have a cardiologist see him. He choked up again.

I read a few days later on his records that he had a positive treadmill, ended up with an angiogram and a stent of one cardiac vessel and went home successfully.

Nothing about this case was remarkable, but everything about it was remarkable. It was a good reminder for me also to fight my nature to rush people and let them tell their story in their own way, because his description of the pain is what made my decision, and it had taken twenty minutes to get that out of him. That is a long time in the Emergency Department.

I think the bottom line of why it hit me at my core was that he was probably a gentleman who had a hard life, who wasn't used to people particularly worrying about him or going out of their way to help him. There are lots of people out there that other people aren't too nice to on a daily basis. And at the end of the day, the whole idea of Emergency Medicine is to treat everyone the same, and that is my favorite thing about it.

The Saddest Case

Another question I get asked is, "What is the saddest thing you have ever seen?" I never directly answer that question, because it is something I can't discuss out loud. I will always remember the names and events of some very rare tragedies. We usually meet for a debriefing after this for our staff as we are all so devastated, but sometimes I can't even force myself to go to those.

There is another thing though which I can describe somewhat, though I don't think I get describe in words the depth of despair it makes me feel, and you will only understand if it has happened in your family.

I saw a woman brought by police. She was a 29-year-old engineer at a high-tech company, which we have an abundance of in our area. She was brought from her apartment, where her neighbors complained that she was acting bizarrely and had flooded her apartment three times.

The story was strange, and I couldn't really put it together. The neighbors thought the patient was mentally ill. I went in to talk with her. She was very pleasant and professional, and dressed nicely. She was clean and well groomed, which is unlike our typical psychiatric patients who often have problems taking care of themselves.

I asked her what had happened today. "Nothing! This is really ridiculous. My water just ran over. There is something wrong with my drains, and I've told them that". That made sense to me, and I began to wonder if she had been falsely accused. I started reading through the police report out loud, slowly. They had interviewed a number of people at the apartments. Her manager described her coming in and out of her door repetitively, slamming the door each time. She had left the water running for hours. It had happened several times, flooding her apartment each time. She was heard to be screaming and praying out loud.

With every sentence I read, she would calmly explain the situation and why they may have thought that. She had been looking for her keys, so was going in and out of her apartment. She had a leaky water valve. She listens to her TV too loud, that must have been what they heard.

I sat and listened to her. Everything made sense, but...there must be something, or why had so many people said the same thing? Finally, I looked calmly at her and asked, "Well, you tell me, is there anything I can do to help you?"

She stared at me for a long time, maybe a minute, maybe longer. She started to speak but her voice wasn't so defensive now, it was almost pleading. "If you could help me, if you know how to...the problem I am having is that, you know at the place I work, someone at work put transistors behind my ears, under my skin. The transistors are under my skin and they are buzzing and telling me things, and it is driving me crazy. I just need to know how to get the transistors out".

I felt a chill down my spine that wasn't shock, it wasn't fear, it was sorrow, that settled into the pit of my stomach. She had schizophrenia. This bright, hard-working, young woman had schizophrenia.

There are some schizophrenics that go on to have relatively normal lives, on medications. I don't see any of those where I work. The ones that I see have a slow, gradual decline, on meds they do OK, then they begin to think the medications are poisoning them (that is part of the disease), stop taking the medications, and descend into the depths of their illness, bouncing in and out of hospitals. Their friends give up on them, their families are in despair. Where I work, we don't see many families that can bear to continue the emotional support though I know that some families do.

A young, promising person in the prime of their life, struck down with mental illness. There are sadder things, but as far as one that fills the heart with despair, that may be the saddest.

Fate

I often fear that I have become too fatalistic on my job. I can predict that the 32-year-old alcoholic who has been in the Emergency Department 17 times this year will not get better, no matter how many times we refer him to alcohol treatment and counseling, or even when we tell him that we fear he will not survive if he continues like this.

I am not surprised when I am called up to resuscitate a 90-year-old patient who fell and broke her hip and was admitted through the Emergency Department three days ago. Ninety-year-olds just so often do not do well with such major surgery.

But, I do know that I am not always right.

We hear the call of the radio, the cackle, "Metro West calling, Code 3". My nurse takes the call but we all listen, 45-year-old, cardiac arrest, shocked three times, now with a pulse, and with a blood pressure 70/40, ETA two minutes. They are coming lights and sirens.

"Well", I think "at least they have a pulse. Maybe we can get him to the cath lab". I call the cardiologist and cath lab to let them know. Time is myocardium as the saying goes.

As we prepare, we see the crew burst through the door, but unexpectedly they are doing CPR. "He arrested again when we got out of the ambulance!" the paramedic says.

As they push him into the room, I see ventricular fibrillation on the monitor, yell "clear", and shock him again, which is now the 4th shock he has received.

Nothing. We shock him again, nothing. One more time, then we see a rhythm. We can feel a pulse but the nurse can't get a blood pressure, which means his blood pressure is less than 60, so we start him on "pressors", medications that increase the blood pressure. I have intubated him and placed him on a ventilator. His EKG now shows an acute anterior myocardial infarction, as we could have predicted.

While we administer medications, the cardiologist arrives. I quickly give the story and they are off to the cath lab.

Though it seemed like he was there 30 minutes to me, I am surprised that the entire event from door to cath lab was 13 minutes., which is pretty good. We try for quick times to protect the heart muscle. However, I do not feel good about this patient. I never saw any movements of his arms or legs, and his pupils were fixed, though that may be from the atropine the paramedics gave him. He had no response at all when I intubated him. He had six shocks in total.

I get back to work, get several things done, then I hear his family is present now in the waiting room. I walk past the room where the patient was on the way to talk with them. It looks like every room after a big resuscitation: Sheets crumpled, blood on the sheet where an IV start was, wrappers from medical equipment on the floor, and equipment out of place.

I walk back to the family room. This is a room where we go to talk to families of critically ill patients when they arrive. It is a rectangular room that is blue and gray, I suppose what are supposed to be calming, colors, a phone, and a Kleenex box. There is a small couch against the far wall, four regular chairs on the right side, and for some reason I have never understood, 6 chairs that are child-size on the left side. It is a bizarre set up, and as the row of children's chairs is an awkward distance of about 3 feet from the adult chairs, which is too far away to sit from the family, plus you would be sitting on a little tiny child's chair which seems odd. So, I usually end up in front of the spouse, half kneeling on the floor, to ask them questions and tell them what is happening. Sometimes the family member is too agitated to sit so they stand or pace, then I stand or pace with them. Every conversation in there is different and you never know what to expect when you walk in.

The hospital pastor is there, which is good. He is sitting with the patient's wife and an 8 year old boy. They all have their heads down praying, but as I look I can see the boy is sobbing. Immediately I have that feeling well up in my throat and eyes, which I hate, and I take a deep breath and tell them the sequence of the Emergency Department events. The fact is though, though families want to know the events, all they really want to know is what is going to happen, and I can't always tell them that. We don't always know what is going to happen ,and this is one of those times. The thing is, they always think you really know, even when you don't. I tell them that I am very worried about the patient, and that I am worried he may have brain damage because of having cardiac arrest, multiple shocks, and a period of having low blood pressure. I try my best to be honest but hopeful, but I do not want to give them false hope.

After we are done, the pastor takes them to the cath lab waiting area. The boy is devastated. I learned later from the nurse that he had been sitting with his dad having ice cream when the dad had sudden cardiac arrest. He hadn't complained of anything before it happened.

That night, about 5 hours later, I call the CCU to see how the patient is doing . Not good. He had a successful angioplasty of a major heart vessel, but neurologically was not waking up at all. In my mind, I review all of his care. Although I know everything went well medically, the normal response if a patient isn't doing well is to question every one of our actions, every medication, and every intervention , and think about if anything should have been done differently. I think of the boy, the look on his face, the fact that he was with his dad when this happened. I feel horrible for the rest of the night.

Later that week, I come to work. Hannah, the nurse involved, yells out to me, "Hey, that patient came down here today". "What patient?" I

52

ask. "That guy that got the six shocks and went to the cath lab". I question her but still really don't believe it. I look up his medical record. On day two of his hospital stay he woke up and had a full neurological recovery. Sometimes I am very happy to be wrong.

Miracle anyone?

I read the nurse's note before I went in. "Chest pain", stated the chief complaint. It noted the pain was worse when the 32-year-old woman took a deep breath. Under Past Medical History, it noted that she had a history of cardiomyopathy, and was on multiple heart medications.

Cardiomyopathy can be caused by a number of illnesses, but in this woman, she had contracted a virus after the birth of her second child. She developed fatigue and severe shortness of breath by the time it was diagnosed two years ago. I reviewed her computerized records, and saw that she had been "listed" for a heart transplant, which meant she was on the waiting-list.

I went to see her, and she described her pain to me. It was right-sided, and worse with a deep breath. It was worse when I pushed on it, which usually implies muscle pain and nothing of concern. Her EKG was normal. Because of her past history though, I thought I had better order a CT angiogram of her chest and an echocardiogram to rule out blood clot or a pericardial effusion.

The CT was normal. The echocardiogram technician came in, and we talked briefly. I told him how poor her heart function was, only 14% on her last echo. He went in the room to do the echo.

After he was done, instead of just leaving a report on the chart like usual, he approached me. "It is a completely normal study", he said. He appeared confused. "Her ejection fraction is up to 55". I stared at him. He was our best echo tech, and I had known him for years. I knew he would not make a mistake on this, but it was hard to believe.

"I pulled her last echo, and this one is completely different. Her contractility is completely normal", he said.

As luck would have it, her cardiologist was actually in the hospital. I contacted him and the echo tech took the study upstairs for him to review.

He called me a short time later. "It is normal", he said. "All of her disease has completely resolved". He was as shocked as I was.

"Well, what should I do?" I asked. She was on five medications for her heart. He had me taper three of her medications and stopped two. He would see her in his office in a few days. He would take her off the transplant list.

I went in to talk to her. She stared at me like I was crazy, as I expected. "Are you sure? " She kept asking. I think she asked it five times. "I don't blame you for not believing it, but it is true. Your cardiologist reviewed the films and I have spoken with him. Your heart function has gone back to normal".

I had never seen this happen before. I have never seen or heard of a patient who is on the heart transplant list have a dramatic improvement like this, and certainly not in the Emergency Department. The patient could not fathom the news at all. Her husband was in the waiting room, and I had him come back so I could talk to him. I felt very odd about stopping heart medications; it is not exactly something I normally do. The funny thing was, none of us acted extremely happy and we didn't celebrate; we talked in hushed tones like it was a secret that we couldn't believe.

I did have to think, it could not have happened to a better person. A young mother, with two small children, who had been having to worry about her own mortality daily. I wondered what she felt like when she walked out of the Emergency Department.

Babies

"Do you ever get to deliver babies?" Is a question I'm frequently asked. What is never suspected, is that in the Emergency Department the last thing we ever want to do is deliver a baby. If a pregnant woman comes to triage we can't get her upstairs to Labor and Delivery fast enough. Everyone I know feels like that; nurses, doctors, techs.

I almost went into OB. It is actually very similar to Emergency Medicine in many ways; you have to think on your feet, it is emotional with rapid decision making, and there are many procedures which I enjoy. In addition, many of us women medical students go through their rotations during their child-bearing years and I think are attracted to OB for that reason. I did more months than required in OB, and loved the deliveries. At that time I felt very comfortable with routine deliveries and knew there was assistance nearby if there was a problem out of my scope.

That was 20 years ago. Now, the thought of deliveries gives me chills. Deliveries are one of those things where everything goes perfectly or everything goes really wrong.

Recently, we heard a yell from the triage area, screaming for a doctor to go out into the parking lot. My partner and I ran out with the delivery bag, and found a woman in the cab of a pickup, her back against her husband, legs spread, with the head already delivered. We gently guided the infant out; well actually, it guided itself out. Ah, thank God, just our kind of delivery. We were both so happy that we stood there smiling idiotically at the baby until the mother suggested we wrap it in a blanket and go inside, so it didn't get hypothermia. It was her 5th baby. We quickly grabbed a blanket and followed her instructions, got the gurney and got them inside.

Another delivery last year occurred in a back of an ambulance, which pulled up lights and sirens during a snow storm. They had called ahead and I ran out to the pull-up where again the baby delivered itself with no problem. The mother was quite sad that dad hadn't made it from work, but otherwise all was well.

I am often asked if patients come in delivering and really don't know they are pregnant. It does happen, and I think there are often many reasons that vary from person to person. Sometimes it is from body habitus, sometimes from denial, but there are some things we probably will never understand.

A chart that I picked up said "Abdominal Pain" as the chief complaint. I saw the patient wheeled back in a wheelchair. She was hunched over with her arms crossed across her stomach, head down. She looked uncomfortable, like she was having pain. I went right in. I often examine patients myself before the nurse comes in, and started talking with the patient.

She complained of abdominal cramping that started four hours before. She was a very nice and polite with my questions, but clearly in pain. I examined her, quickly listening to her heart and lungs, then examined her stomach. Immediately I had my suspicious as she was quite thin but her very lower portion of her abdomen was tender and protuberant.

I then set her up for a pelvic examination, and quickly realized why her upper abdomen wasn't that large: The baby was already crowning, meaning the head was visible at the vagina. My first thought was, "Jesus Christ". My second thought was, "I'm in the room by myself." I called out to the nurse as I gently started applying pressure to the head. The nurse walked in, then literally turned around as fast as she could and walked back out when she saw what was happening. She didn't say one word.

I started talking to the patient soothingly and explained what was happening to her. She was crying and clearly in distress both physically and emotionally as she contracted. Now the room filled with staff as my nurse had alerted everyone, and I had Respiratory Therapy, three nurses, a tech and another doctor. A heated bassinette was in the room now. I gently delivered the first shoulder, then the second shoulder, and the baby slipped out. At this time the NICU folks had arrived, we are always glad to see them, and they finished everything up.

I went up to the mom's head area now, and started talking with her. She was amazingly calm now, but scared. I hadn't even asked her if someone had come with her but did so now. "My boyfriend, but I don't want you to tell him anything" she cried.

"OK", I said, but what do you want me to tell him?" "I don't know, just send him away". I had the triage nurse put him in the family room. I went out later and told him that she was ill and needed to be admitted, and that he should go. He refused to leave though, and wanted to see her. I told him I would send someone out later.

What I heard later is that he refused to leave, and eventually she agreed to see him and told him. I don't know any of the rest of the story. I don't know if it was his, if they suspected she was pregnant, or if they wanted the baby. They both seemed like very nice, normal people. It was just one of those things where you knew there was a lot more to the story then you would ever know, and that you weren't ever going to find out.

A very distressing delivery occurred several years ago when I was called out to the bathroom in our lobby. I ran through the triage doors and into the bathroom, which I had never been in before. The nurse told me there was a girl with abdominal pain sitting on the toilet. She was screaming in pain, sweating, and was in obvious distress.

"Let's get her off the toilet, get a gurney!", I said to the staff, and we gently lifted her up. As we helped her stand I looked into the toilet to see an infant dangling by the umbilical cord into the toilet water. I quickly lifted it, and as I cradled it in my arms gave it mouth-to-mouth respirations as I had no Ambu ventilation bag with me. We heard a small gurgling sound as we rushed them both back to a room.

We began aggressively resuscitating the baby once in the back, and the NICU team had come down in record time to help us. They did an excellent job of placing an IV in the umbilicus and intubating the child. As they did this, I turned my attention to the mom. She could talk now but was very tearful. She was 17-years-old, and she was completely distraught. I asked her if I could call her parents and she tearfully told me they were in Europe and she couldn't reach them.

That one still bothers me to this day when I think about it, this poor girl must have labored at home for hours before arriving in our Emergency Department, and headed straight to the bathroom without even checking in to the triage nurse because she was in so much pain when she got there. Thank God, the infant did OK. I never learned the whole story with the mother either, or even when her parents arrived, I just know that she was admitted upstairs and that was the last I heard of her. That is a rough way to start a new life for both of them.

What do Flashlights and Carrots have in common?

"Foreign Body" read the triage note at the top of my chart. The nurse's notes were missing as I grabbed the chart. It had been a busy night shift. Oh well, I would just go in to the patient's room and not keep them waiting as I searched for the nurse's notes.

I entered the room to find a gentleman with gray hair and a muscular build. Right away I got a strange vibe from the room, he seemed very hostile. "I see from the triage note that you are having problems with a foreign body?" I asked .

"Yes, it's in my ass, that's why I'm here, and I don't want to go through the story again" he said angrily. He told me it was a carrot and had been there for over 6 hours, and he had tried everything to get it out. He was very angry and expressed to me that he couldn't stay long in the Emergency Department, he needed to have it taken out right away.

I told him we would set everything up and give him conscious sedation to remove it. This made him agitated; he didn't want any medications, "Just get it out". I tried to discuss this with him as it would be quite painful to remove it but he declined.

With a nurse and technician in assistance, I had the patient lay on his side. I could feel the tip of the carrot, but I could also see that his rectum was very irritated with dried blood present from his own attempts to remove it. I gently inserted some small forceps and could grasp the carrot, but as it had been in there quite a while and the tip was pointing down, it would just break off. After several attempts, he was now having a small amount of bleeding which was making it harder. "Hurry up! Just get it out!" he yelled at me.

I tried several other maneuvers without success, and he unleashed his anger again on me. At this point, which was about 2 in the morning, I had enough. "OK, I am sorry it is taking so long, but the fact is, I didn't put it up there, and after your attempts to get it out you have swelling and bleeding. I'm doing the best that I can", I stated.

He proceeded to tell me that he had to pick up his wife at the airport this morning. "You aren't going to make it.", I stated firmly. "This needs to come out, and we need to sedate you now". Finally, he agreed.

With sedation, we were able to gently work the large carrot out and place it on a silver tray, where it would go to pathology (all objects removed from the human body must go to the lab).

Although he couldn't pick up his wife, I had a tech call her and say he was in the Emergency Department with stomach pain. She arrived to pick him up later that morning. Hopefully, the pathology report didn't show up on the bill, but he did leave happier than when he came according to the nurse.

I had a very pleasant gentleman come in a number of years ago. I went to see him before the nurse because she was busy in another patient's room. The patient shook my hand warmly, and when I asked what brought him in, he said, "Well, I put a flashlight in my rectum, and I can't get it out". He then apologized profusely. He explained that his wife had died a number of years ago, and he did this for sexual release. He was the most delightful man, and very patient with our efforts. It took a while as it was so wide and slippery, but eventually we succeeded in its removal.

This was a nice change because the one thing I don't like is when people lie about how it got in there. If you have a light bulb in your rectum, or a screwdriver or a vibrator, please do not tell us you were assaulted and someone put it up there or that you fell on it in the shower. If we had a dollar for every time we heard that one…that is why I appreciated the honesty so much of the gentleman with the flashlight. I completely don't judge anyone for their sexual practices, but I must say it kind of adds insult to injury when I need to dig something out when they won't tell me the truth or are screaming at me about it.

We do take care of a lot of women who get a tampon stuck and can't get it out. They are mortally embarrassed, but I will have to say this isn't even on our radar screen as something embarrassing. It's very common and completely understandable. Usually the triage nurse will call me, and they put the patient in a little private room at the end of the hall. I go in myself with just a speculum and a little ring forceps. One minute and we are done. I don't make the patients wait for discharge paperwork as they just want to get out of there as fast as they can at that point, so I try to make it easy for them.

Other Foreign Bodies

More typically, the foreign bodies we see are objects placed in the nose, ears, or mouth by children. I always get a real kick out of these and they are usually challenging and interesting to remove.

Beads up the nose are very common and usually quite easy to remove. Beads in the ears can be challenging but are also common.

One little 4—year-old I recently took care of came in with a rock in his ear. He had found the rock on his playground at pre-school. He was a very cooperative little guy and I removed it easily. We were always trained to then check the other ear, which I did and found a rock in it also. After I removed it, I asked him, "Why did you put the rocks in there?"

I usually ask this question just for my personal entertainment to be honest. "Because my ears have been hurting so much", he said sadly. I then took a good look at his ear drums to find them bright red and infected. He had placed the rocks in an effort to help the pain, poor little guy. We gave him some Tylenol and placed him on antibiotics.

Another two-year-old recently put a bead up his nose. His mom spoke only Spanish, and his sister, who was seven and adorable, spoke excellent English. I tried to use our Spanish phone translator as I set up my equipment to take out the bead, but the two-year-old was screaming so loud it drowned out our conversation. The seven-year-old happily translated for me, her voice rising above the din.

I went ahead and grabbed the instruments I need and started, though the nurse couldn't come help me hold the baby down as she was busy. From looking at the mom, I knew she would be able to help me hold down this kid; sometimes you can just tell. Some parents just can't do it, they will try but then the kid's arm will fly up and hit you, or the legs are kicking and they can't manage them. This mom, within a minute of me asking, had the kid pinned to the gurney and he couldn't move a muscle.

The sister held his legs. They held him perfectly still despite his protests, and I used my favorite instrument, a tiny wire loop. I slipped it gently and slowly behind the bead and then pulled it out. With the mom holding and the sister translating, it took us about two minutes total. Afterwards, the seven-year-old hugged me, and the mom was so relieved, saying "gracias, gracias", over and over. My favorite case of the night, easily. Sometimes it is the little things that make your day.

And More Foreign Bodies

My partner and I were both standing at the desk working. The unit secretary placed a new chart in the rack, which read, "Rectal Foreign Body" as the chief complaint. "I'll see it," my male partner volunteered when he saw the patient was a man. "Thanks, I'm sure the patient would prefer it," I said.

The patient was to go into room 5, and several seconds later we saw the volunteer walking the patient into room 5. With him were his wife and daughter, who was about 10. "Well, that's a new twist,", my partner said. " I've never had a rectal foreign body patient bring his family with him". We looked at each other, both shocked.

I got to work checking on a patient, but when I went back to the desk, the nurse said, "Dr. Gregg needs you in room 5". I wasn't that surprised as often we help each other remove rectal foreign bodies. They can be very difficult to remove, and sometimes an extra pair of hands is helpful. Sometimes one doctor can hold the anoscope, while the other doctor holds the forceps trying to remove the culprit foreign body, or sometimes, with the patient in fetal position, one doctor will gently push on the patient's abdomen to push the foreign body down while the other physician, positioned at the rectum, tries to grasp it as it descends.

I headed into room 5. When I got there, the patient was positioned on his back, with his legs spread and in the stirrups, as one would position a patient for a pelvic exam. As I approached from behind Dr. Gregg, I saw that he was applying gentle pressure to remove a long, thick, white object from the patient's rectum. I looked closer—it looked like a giant worm. It's white, glistening body was emerging from the patient's rectum. It was thick, white, and with somewhat thickened sides. My partner was applying gentle traction on it to try and remove it without breaking it. "Can you assist me here?" he said calmly. I grasped the end with an instrument so that he could move his hands up closer to the part of the worm protruding closer at the patient's rectum, and he continued pulling. The worm continued slowly coming out. There was approximately two feet of it coming when I walked in, and slowly, gradually, it elongated.

By the time it had completely emerged, it was over 4 feet in length. The nurse put it in a large basin to send to the lab. It looked like it came out in one piece, thankfully.

My partner and I later talked, completely shocked. He said he didn't really need my help, he just wanted to call me in to see it because he was so amazed and wanted someone else to see it.

It turned out later that the patient had been eating fish out of the Willamette River, and somehow picked up this giant tapeworm, we thought, from the fish. The night he was seen, he felt something emerging from his rectum, which is when he decided to come in. He had no idea that he had worms. He was given "anti-worm" medicine later to be sure he had no other worms or eggs in his intestines.

That is the only case I have seen like that ever, and it still gives me pause when I am about to eat fish.

New Diagnoses

By far, the least favorite and most surreal part of my job is that very rare occurrence when I find something awful on a CT scan which shows a patient has cancer. This happens probably three or four times a year. Often it is completely unexpected.

Many patients think they have cancer when they arrive. In our society we all worry we have cancer so every ache and pain makes us fear the worst. However, cancer actually very rarely causes pain in the early stages. I often see patients who think they have cancer, but instead have gallstones, kidney stones, or an ovarian cyst.

Unfortunately, the opposite scenario can occur. I recently had a very pleasant 45-year-old mechanical engineer who presented feeling that he must have a pinched nerve in his neck because his arm wasn't working right. He was having troubles with his laptop and playing the piano. The entire story worried me but more so for stroke. I ordered a scan of his head and was very dismayed when the radiologist called to tell me there was a large brain tumor. After 10 minutes to mentally prepare myself, and leaving my phone at the desk so that I wouldn't be interrupted, I told this gentleman who woke up this morning with a normal life that he had a brain tumor. His wife sat by his side, holding his hand with tears running down her face. The patient didn't act shocked or even upset. I think that deep down sometimes people know something is really wrong. He was admitted where he underwent surgery and started chemotherapy.

These cases completely devastate all of us caring for the patient as well. One recent case though was not what I expected. I had an elderly female, 86, who came in with some abdominal pain. She had a past history of uterine cancer, but when I questioned her about it I found she had not seen her doctor for follow-up as suggested. "I hate doctors! No offense", she laughed. She was a very pleasant, funny, delightful lady. I ended up doing a CT scan of her abdomen and pelvis which showed multiple large masses. Again, after having a few moments to gather my thoughts, I went in to talk with her.

She had been alone on arrival as she lived by herself at home, so I was surprised when I walked in now that she had multiple family members including two small grandchildren present. I sat down next to her and explained what we saw on the CT scan. I told her it was bad news, and that the radiologist and I thought that the masses were probably cancerous tumors. "I am so sorry, I wish there was anything else I could tell you, but I want to be completely honest with you", I said.

She grabbed my hand tightly, closed her eyes for a second, then opened them and smiled. "Don't you feel bad for one minute", she said. "I've had a great life and have enjoyed every minute. That isn't going to change. I'm 86, I'm not going to live forever", she said in a strong voice.

I started to discuss specialists, referrals, etc. She stopped me and said, "No, I really do hate hospitals. There is no way I'm getting chemo or surgery at my age." She explained her rationale. She had seen friends go through it, and that she just wanted to enjoy her family. Her family gathered around her, touching her, rubbing her back. Her small grandson piped in, "Grandma, do you want to play with my Matchbox truck?" Everyone laughed, and his mother said he could tell something was wrong and wanted to help. I think she was absolutely right. Some kids really do have a 6th sense. It also broke the tension in the room. We discussed pain management, hospice, and the family talked about how they would help her.

She refused to stay in the hospital even for the night, and went home with her family. The phrase "Grace under pressure", kept coming to mind the whole night. Some people really are class acts, even when told the worst news about themselves that they will ever receive.

Basketball Practice

"You're getting a seizure patient in room 42", the charge nurse told me. I was working pediatrics, and getting a kid with a seizure was a very common occurrence, usually caused by fevers. I continued my charting, then looked up to see the ambulance crew rushing in. The first thing I noticed is that one of them was sweating and appeared very concerned. He was a great paramedics so I approached quickly, knowing something was really wrong.

"Fever and rash. He had the flu the last three days, then mom noticed a rash this morning. He got Benadryl before mom went to work. Dad went in around 1pm and couldn't wake him up". In front of me was a 17-year-old, who was struggling and combative on the stretcher. Both paramedics were trying to hold him down as they arrived. The paramedic was sweating because he had been struggling with this big strong kid the whole way in.

On his skin, the rash that we all fear: Purple blotches, covering his skin. Meningococcus. Portland, where I live, has had one of the highest meningococcal rates in the country for unknown reasons. There is an immunization now but the immunization doesn't help with the strain we have and we still see it.

The paramedics had placed an IV en route, but the patient had pulled it out. Two nurses immediately went to work and got an IV. Another nurse ran to get medications and we paralyzed him quickly and intubated him, all within about five minutes. The father was in the room and I tried to explain things as we went, but I was really worried about this kid. We started steroids and antibiotics.

The steroids are important because when meningococcal bacteria are swimming around in our blood stream, and then we start an antibiotic, all those bacteria lyse or "pop" open from the antibiotic, and release toxins into the blood stream and spinal cord which do a great deal of damage to the tissues. Patients with meningococcal disease, if they live, can lose their arms and legs from tissue damage. Their adrenal glands can turn into one big blood clot.

We are supposed to start the steroids and wait 30 minutes for the antibiotics; I can usually make it about 5 minutes because I want the antibiotics in quickly and can't stand the wait. Everything was started on this kid, he now had three IV's, steroids, antibiotics, was intubated and on a ventilator, and was receiving medications to support his blood pressure. Report had been called to the ICU. His blood work was coming back, and showed that his blood clotting functions were very abnormal, a bad sign.

I had a conference with dad outside of the room before the patient went to ICU. "He'll be fine, right?" Dad asked me. I told him I was very concerned the patient wouldn't be fine. This kid was extremely sick and I told dad that I was worried he would have serious complications and could die. I went through all of the treatments he had received and what we would be doing.

"But he'll be fine, right?" Dad asked again, very concerned. Was he hearing anything I said? I repeated everything, talked about meningococcus, the very high death rate associated with it, why we were putting him in the unit, that we were giving him medications to support his blood pressure.

"My wife is calling", he said as he looked at his cell phone. His voice was shaking I noticed. When he lifted the cell phone to answer his hands were shaking so much he could barely hold it. "I can tell her that he'll be fine, right?" I told him I would talk to her and told her my concerns. She would be at the hospital in 30 minutes.

As they wheeled him out of the room to the ICU, dad approached me again. "So you think he'll be OK, right?" he asked, taking my hand.

"I don't know", is all I meant to say. I don't know why, and it kills me to this day, but I said, "Yes, I think he'll be OK". I think it was the desperation, the look on the dad's face, the shaking in his voice. I don't know why I said it and I regretted it immediately. I went home that night feeling sick and feeling angry at myself for saying that.

Two days later, I checked on him in the ICU. He had woken up and was doing great. I talked to the dad. "Boy, I was so upset in the ER. What a complete nightmare for all of us,", the dad said. "The only thing that got me though it was you were so positive and thought he would be OK". Great. The nurses told me the next week that the patient and dad stopped off in the Emergency Department to talk to everyone but I was gone. He said to say thanks.

I viewed this as one giant reprieve. I always try to tell the exact truth and what I'm thinking and not give false hope, and to this day I still don't know why I said what I did.

***Lie Detector ***

One of my favorite partners, who has been in practice for 30 years, often says that the technology we need most in the Emergency Department is a lie detector. He is only partially joking. The fact is, we are very often lied to in the Emergency Department, for a variety of reasons.

We all have taken care of countless teenagers who have never had sex but have a positive pregnancy test; patients with rectal foreign bodies who "fell on it" (a light bulb? A screwdriver?), or were assaulted and someone put it up there; or who had "just two drinks" but their blood alcohol is sky-high.

My first distinct memory of a patient lying to me occurred when I was a resident in the Emergency Department. I responded to a trauma in the Emergency Department. We had already received a radio report that it was a patient who was shot with an arrow. We did not know until he arrived that the patient had been shot through the head.

The patient arrived, sitting up on a gurney, with the arrow going straight through the middle of his forehead. The tip was not protruding through the back.

"I was just walking through the forest, and someone shot me!", the patient said. He did not know the assailants. The paramedics and police arrived with the patient, but the patient could not describe the assailants to them either.

His Emergency Department care consisted only of an examination, IV's, pain medications, and antibiotics, then off he went to the OR for removal by the neurosurgeons, utilizing special x-ray imaging studies to be sure they didn't injure the arteries.

That night we all talked about this poor patient, being shot while just out for a walk, straight through the head. We wondered if he was mistaken for a deer, who knew?

The next morning, I opened up the newspaper. There was a picture of the patient, on the front page. The story went on to describe how the patient was out with his friends, drinking. He bet his friends that they could not shoot an apple off of his head. He got an apple, stood up against a tree, and gave his friend his bow and arrow. And that is how he got shot straight through the head.

The patient did well and left the hospital with no neurological complications.

More recently, I took care of a young woman who had been found by her regular doctor to have a sky-high blood pressure. It was about 250/150 if I remember correctly. She had no history of medical problems at all, and no family history of hypertension. She was a very lovely young woman, a college student.

I asked her about substance abuse, and she denied it.

I did a CT scan of her brain , blood work, and I ordered a urine. I started her on medications for her blood pressure.

The nurse told me she hadn't gotten the urine yet because the patient had gone right before she got there. That should have been a red flag for me.

I got busy doing other things, then went to check on her. Her blood pressure had not improved much at all, and her blood work was normal. They still hadn't gotten the urine because she accidentally flushed it. I felt that I had to admit her because of her blood pressure.

I talked with her again. "OK, so you are sure you haven't used any drugs at all?"

"No, absolutely not", she said.

"You're not going to throw me under the bus on this, right?" I asked. "I've already told the hospitalist and cardiologist that I consulted that you don't use."

She promised me again that she hadn't used. I admitted her upstairs without waiting on the urine. Two hours later, I checked the computer. Her cocaine was positive.

Even though I shouldn't be surprised by much at this point, I was still a little surprised. You really can't tell by talking to people sometimes.

Narcotic Dispensers

One of our charge nurses, who has worked at our Emergency Department for 30 years, keeps saying if we just put a narcotic dispenser in the lobby it would cut down our visits by 50%. Our staff often makes jokes like this to deal with the constant stress of this problem, but the reality of narcotic abuse is devastating.

There are definitely patients who need to be on chronic narcotics. Patients with cancer pain, patients with peripheral neuropathy, elderly who have chronic pain; narcotics can make their pain at least tolerable. There is clearly a role for chronic narcotics for some indications.

We, as medical professionals, often get patients started on the path to narcotic abuse. Someone comes in with an ankle injury, for example, and receives Vicodin. Their ankle may not recover rapidly, and they see their own physician in follow-up who gives them more Vicodin. In some patients, that is enough of a trigger that their bodies begin craving it. It can happen amazingly fast, and often I don't believe that patients are warned about narcotics when they receive them.

On top of this, there was a big push in the last ten years to treat pain more aggressively. It is definitely true that physicians used to not be as aggressive as they should in treating pain, particularly in children, and in cases where pain medications are absolutely necessary such as cancer pain. However, this led to everything from minor lacerations and sore throats that used to be treated with Tylenol now being treated with narcotics. Narcotic abuse has been around forever, but now it has became a problem of epic proportions. This year in my state, prescription drug deaths overtook recreational drug deaths (cocaine, heroin, etc) as a cause of death. More people even died of prescription drug overdoses than motor vehicle accidents.

Narcotics are now widely available on the internet. Almost everyone has received a "spam" email for Vicodin at some time. I don't know how that problem will ever be reigned in.

There are red flags for identifying patients who may be abusing narcotics, and who are frequenting Emergency Departments and "Doctor Shopping". Before I go see a patient, I typically review their records to know their diagnoses, medications, and allergies. If a patient has been in the Emergency Department, for example, ten times in the last year and received narcotics every time for a variety of reasons, it is concerning that there may be a problem. It is amazing how often this happens.

When a physician goes in to see these patients, there are often patterns. They are usually very ingratiating at first to the physician, complimenting them, and thanking them profusely. The story of why they are there often doesn't make complete sense. For example, they hurt their wrist, often from a fall on the stairs or at work, but there are no signs of trauma.

Often these patients bring a child with them to the Emergency Department, even if it is in the middle of the night. I've never really understood that one but it is a recurrent theme. There is also a frequent story about they injured themselves while helping an elderly family move into a care facility or moving out the belongings of a dead family member. I just had one patient who had used both stories about his dad on prior visits, after he came to the Emergency Department hunched over and holding his back. When he told me he was helping his dad move I reminded him that last time he was there he told me his dad died. He dressed and quickly left, not hunched over anymore and not holding his back, and declined my offer for a drug treatment program.

When you look at the records, often these patients have had multiple visits for car accidents in the past; sometimes an unbelievable number, like 20 or 30. While possible, it is unlikely, especially if they have never been found to have any documented injuries.

I always am completely honest; after a work-up I discuss with the patients that the x-rays or whatever tests are ordered are normal. The fact is, these patients have a disease just like any other patient, and you have to be compassionate towards that and at least offer drug treatment. The patient will usually then request narcotics, and I will discuss I am concerned because they have had 34 visits this year and received narcotics each visit, and I discuss that I don't feel comfortable prescribing narcotics. I discuss the risks of narcotics such as addiction, respiratory depression, even death. I offer to treat with non-narcotic alternatives.

This is when it usually hits the fan. They become angry, accuse me of a variety of things such as not caring about them, not knowing what I am doing, etc. I offer non-narcotic therapies but these are usually refused. Usually at this point the patient storms off. Sometimes security has to be called because they become violent or threatening.

I always worry about not treating pain in a patient who really has a painful condition, but when you have this situation re-played over 10 times a shift I fear I will become calloused.

I took care of a lovely 25-year-old girl several years ago who had a history of frequent Emergency Department visits for pain complaints. She was now seen with neck pain after awakening. I listened to her story, and examined her carefully. I felt it was muscle pain, and her story wasn't concerning for anything more serious. "When I get something like this, they usually give me a medication that starts with a P, I can't remember the name…" "Percocet?" I suggested. "Yes, that's it. I think if I just have a few of those I can rest so I can go to work tomorrow."

I took a deep breath. "You now, I am worried you may have a problem. You have been here 16 times in the last two years for pain

complaints, and have gotten narcotics every visit. They are really ad-
dictive and I wonder if we have caused you a problem."

I leaned back and waited for the storm. I looked at her, and saw
her eyes fill with tears. She went on to explain that she knew she was
addicted, but as soon as she ran out she went to different clinics and
Emergency Departments to get refills. She had been to every hospital
in our city. Her mother had also been a prescription drug addict. She
was so ashamed; so remorseful. It is the first and only time I have ever
had someone admit to this in 20 years. I thanked her for her honesty
and we talked about treatment options. Our social worker was able to
line her up with a program. I don't know how she did.

When I was in residency, we had a hard core drug-seeker come
into the Emergency Department. I truly don't recall our entire interaction, but I did make it clear to him he would not receive narcotics. He
became very angry and had to be escorted out of the Emergency Department by security. This had happened with him a number of times.
Several hours later, I was walking into the break room when he suddenly appeared in front of me in the dark hallway, and demanded that
I write him a prescription. My heart jumped into my throat, and I could
barely get words out, but I told him I would go get my prescription
pad and be right back. I notified security and they escorted him out. I
felt lucky that he hadn't had a knife and that it ended as it did.

When we have patients who visit the Emergency Department
over and over, for less than what are considered significant reasons,
they are labeled "frequent fliers". Unfortunately, almost always these
patients are seeking narcotics. Narcotic addiction in this country is an
enormous problem as anyone who works in the Emergency Department will attest.

However, every now and then we will get a look into these patient's lives. One of our frequent fliers who presented for back pain
came into the Emergency Department. He had had back surgeries
years prior, and often presented with acute back pain, but all further

tests and imaging studies had been normal for 15 years. I had seen him once before myself, but on the computer I noted that he had been seen over 100 times in the Emergency Department in the last 4 years. When I went in, his wife was with him. I had not met her before. After talking with the patient and examining him, I went out and spoke with his doctor. "DO NOT give him narcotics,", his doctor said. He has been going from ER to ER. This is the fourth call I've had this week. I'm terminating him as a patient. I have been giving him six Percocets a day, but the agreement was he wouldn't keep going into ER's, and he is still doing it and lying about it" he said, obviously frustrated.

I went back in the room and talked with the patient and his wife. The patient became angry, as expected. The wife walked out of the room and asked that I follow her.

Once in the hall, she told me that she didn't know what to do. Not only was the patient going from Emergency Department to Emergency Department, he was actually buying narcotics on the street. She said at home he didn't act like he had back pain, he could do all of his usual activities, but once in the Emergency Department he would complain of severe pain.

I talked with her and then the patient. I offered to place him in Chemical Dependency for treatment but of course he refused, and we can't make patients go there against their will.

I do not have a happy ending for this story. The patient is still in a similar situation. He is on disability for back pain, and still shows up in various Emergency Departments from time to time trying to get narcotics. It would be interesting medically to know all of the places he had gone. That is impossible though as hospitals aren't allowed to share records without a patient's permission.

It is just overall a truly heartbreaking situation. The patients truly have some type of pain, be it physical or psychogenic; the doctors they see often perpetuate the problem, and the family is often help-less to stop it.

I would estimate that approximately ten percent of patients seen on a daily basis in the Emergency Department have a substance abuse problem, and I think most doctors would place that at a higher figure. I do not have answers for it, I wish I did, but all we can do is try to help the patient as best as we can, which is often not the type of help they want.

I have had several friends who cite the narcotic-seeking patients as a major reason in why they retired early from the Emergency De-partment. They are often desperate patients who will do everything in their power to get narcotics. Most health care providers want to help people, so it sets up an internal conflict for the health care providers.

To compound the problem, there are very few substance abuse treatment facilities for the patients who really want help. It really is an overwhelming problem with no end in site.

There are patients who sell the narcotics they receive in the Emer-gency Department on the streets. The press has recently documented several cases of this. We have had deaths of teenagers from narcotics that came out of the Emergency Department and medical offices for another patient, who then sold them to a teenager.

The desperation that narcotics create for patients is a tragic situ-ation. It is an endemic problem that truly does not seem to be getting any better, especially with the onset of use of Oxycontin which has created an entire new generation of narcotic abusers.

Narcotic abuse will always be a problem in the Emergency De-partment. While it is our job to treat pain in patients with acute condi-tions, it is also our job to identify this, be compassionate towards the patients, and try to get them the help they need. It is a disease, just like any other medical condition. As a professional, it wears you down beyond belief. Most of us went into the profession to help others, and to tell people "No" is often a very unfulfilling but necessary part of our jobs. It is often considered patronizing and cruel by some, but as a professional you must know all of the consequences of narcotics and try to help the patient, even if it is not how they want to be helped.

Nose for the Job

After you work in the Emergency Department for a while, you like to think you have a "sixth sense" about what is going on with patients. Of course you can't always tell, it is often the first and only time you will meet that patient.

This works both ways. Sometimes I'll have a patient come in with some complaint I don't understand, like "my left ankle has been hurting all day and it is swollen". I look at the ankle and it looks completely normal. The patient is walking around normally. They don't remember any injury to the ankle. X-rays are normal. OK, I'm really stumped now. Then, at the time of discharge, they will ask me for a note for the last six days off work. So, they had to miss work for whatever reason, and now they need a note. This happens not infrequently. After a while, you learn to ask more questions up front if the story doesn't really make sense.

Once I had a child, about two, who had a cold with a mild stuffy nose. The child otherwise looked great and was eating chips out of a bag (from the vending machine in our lobby I am ashamed to say, I still can't believe we have it). The child had no fever, no ear pain, no vomiting, no rash. The mother seemed fairly upset from the minute she got there, and I couldn't tell what her concern was. Finally, I asked her. "Well, I'm in the middle of a custody battle, and her dad had her for the last two days. I want a note that she has this cold and he didn't take her to the doctor's office or get her checked." This made me quite uncomfortable, as I felt that 99% of parents would not bring their child in for this complaint, and I didn't feel that the dad had been negligent. I declined to write her a letter as she wanted but told her she could always request the medical records later if she wanted.

On the other hand, sometimes patients come in and completely minimize their complaint. This is usually because a family member forces them to come in.

Several years ago I took care of a pleasant, somewhat heavy, 50-year-old man. He was wearing a football jersey and jeans. Oregon Ducks fan. Very nice guy. He said he was there because he felt "a little weak on the left". "I just want to get it checked out, but I think I'm fine," he volunteered. He had a history of high blood pressure and hypertension.

His examination was completely normal. I ordered blood work and a CT of his head. To my surprise, the CT showed evidence of four small strokes that had occurred in the past (often recent strokes don't show up on plain CT scans, as it takes a certain amount of time for the brain changes to show up. These days we usually do an MRI or a CT angiogram to look at the arteries if we feel there is an acute event).

I went in to talk to him after getting the CT report. I had already ordered his bed, writing out the order even as the radiologist was giving me report. It was a slam dunk admission.

I told the patient his findings. "OK doc, thanks. But I'm not going to stay, I will follow up with my doctor though." I was dumbstruck. I started pressuring him, telling him he was most likely having a small stroke today given his CT findings of having prior infarcts (areas in the brain which didn't get enough blood supply). I told him he could have a large stroke or even die if he left, and that he absolutely needed to stay. "I understand, thanks, but I've really got to go." He started walking out. I stood there in shock as he walked out the door. Usually patients will at least talk it over with me, but this guy was just out the door.

I went grabbed the chart and dialed the phone number on it. Fortunately, his wife answered the phone. I introduced myself, told her I couldn't talk about the patient until she got there, but that I needed him back in the Emergency Department right now.

"Oh my gosh", she said. "I made him come in, but he wants to leave to go to the Duck's game with his friends. They are all driving down together, and he promised me he would come get checked first."

"I will have him back there in five minutes." She said. I knew she would.

Sure enough, a very short time afterwards, a triage nurse walked the sheepish patient back to the same room. I went in to talk to him. I told him I would call the neurologist and get him admitted, and he agreed. I also told him we would put the TV on the local college game, but he was still grumpy about that and said it wouldn't be the same. He hadn't missed a game in 10 years, this was the first one.

My usual goal in these situations is to wait until I turn away from the patient before rolling my eyes, but I broke my rule in this case. I had just put a lot of work as well as anxiety into getting this patient admitted, and he was whining and complaining about missing the game, even though he could watch it on TV. And I will add, I am a big football fan, also, but come on.

I often tell patients that there is a study that men who are married live longer, but women who are married have shorter life spans. I can't count the times that I have had a wife drag her husband in because she knows something is wrong, and I will have to say that 90% of the time their assessment is correct.

Women also often minimize their symptoms. The classic case I see of this is with kidney stones. I've always said I am going to do a study about women presenting with kidney stones. Not to sound sexist, but we often know a male kidney stone patient is present when they are in the lobby. They are writhing, screaming in pain, and are rushed back (appropriately so) for an IV and immediate narcotics.

I have had women who have sat patiently in the waiting room with the words "flank pain" or "back pain" on the chart, stating their pain is "3/10", and when they get back and I talk to them, they calmly tell me it is the worse pain they've ever had. "Worse than childbirth?" I ask. "Oh, yes". If yes is the answer, I am 100% correct in diagnosing a kidney stone.

I don't know if it is different anatomy or different pain threshold, but there is a difference.

And although these situations are interesting and sometimes funny, the concern is that we are trying to judge what is wrong with a patient by their estimation of their pain and their behavior, when the fact is that we don't know the patient, don't know their pain threshold, and could make a big "miss" by underestimating someone's pain scale.

I have heard one of my partner's, a prior Special Ops guy in the military, when patients say their pain is a 10/10 with a complaint say, such as, an ingrown toenail. "OK", he will say, "so to me, a 10/10 is some-one pouring gas on you and setting you on fire". Somehow I think he may have seen that somewhere based on the way he says it.

The opposite also occurs, and I've had patients with an obvi-ously severely painful injury, such as a nail through their foot, say that their pain is a 2/10. I can't help but wonder what they would consider a 10/10.

I think the main goal has to be a high index of suspicion, and although the pain scale we use now, 1 to 10, is important, you have to have a nose for that situation where the patient is either overreporting or underreporting their pain, and that is part of why medicine really is an art and not a science in the Emergency Department.

***Happy Customers ***

I was just walking down a hall when I saw a boy who was a tall, gangly kid taken into a room. He was holding his hand over his mouth, which was bleeding. He had no one with him except the triage nurse. I walked in and found out that he had been walking to football practice after school, when he walked by a person from the golf team. The golfer took a big swing back, and had knocked out this kid's upper four teeth. I immediately asked if he had the teeth, which he did, in his pocket. We retrieved them and put them in a solution which we have for knocked-out teeth. I asked the nurse to place an IV and gave him pain medications and antibiotics. The kid was a real trooper, not complaining, but obviously in pain.

At that point, his parents arrived. The father immediately started yelling at me, asking me why I wasn't doing anything. I actually recognized the father from an activity I had seen him at before. The mother didn't say anything but sat with an angry expression on her face. Neither said anything to their son. I explained to him what we had done, and that I had ordered a CT scan to assess his jaw and face for fractures. He didn't calm down, and threatened litigation if there was not a good outcome.

Although annoying, you can't let stuff like this get to you. No one (well, almost no one) is ever happy to be in the Emergency Department, though this guy was a little over the top. It was a little frustrating that I felt like we had seen the patient immediately and had been doing everything possible and they were still unhappy, but so be it.

I then had the tray set up and immediately and carefully reimplanted his teeth. The teeth sucked up perfectly into the sockets, though they were clearly unstable. I lost myself in the work and forgot for a few minutes about the dad.

The CT showed a fracture of his maxilla but not severe. While the patient was in CT, I found out the name of his orthodontist from his mom, who agreed to see him on a Friday at 3 pm no less (this was a true miracle, and has never happened before or since). I repaired the large laceration he had on his upper lip, and told the parents to take him immediately to the orthodontist. The orthodontist, a great guy, called me later to tell me that he had put braces on the kid to stabilize the teeth.

I saw the kid (at a social event) six months later. The dad was actually pretty civil and even pleasant. All of the teeth had "taken" and looked perfect.

What would the outcome be if the teeth hadn't taken? We will never know, but this does illustrate the classic situation of a very angry family who will not be happy with anything less than perfection, which cannot always happen. But all you can do is stay calm, do your best, and hope that they see you are trying everything to take care of their family member.

Families

Speaking to families is part of the job in the Emergency Department. Family members are always involved with every patient. You can get very helpful information from them, they will bring in the patient's medication bottles when there is a question, and they are involved with every decision along the way in most cases.

Recently I had a Code Blue patient brought in, on Christmas Day. The patient had been found unresponsive on Christmas morning. The paramedics were called and attempted resuscitation, intubating the patient and administering multiple rounds of ACLS medications. They had found the patient initially with no heart rhythm, then got a rhythm on the monitor but no pulse. When they arrived and told me that I was a little surprised that they brought the patient in. Often they will "call" these in the field, pronouncing the patient dead, as the chance for resuscitation is so dismal. This patient had no pulse for over 40 minutes, which means that even if he were resuscitated the chances of brain death are incredibly high.

The patient had a history of high cholesterol and hypertension, and was slightly obese. Everything sounded like a massive heart attack. We ran the code for another 15 minutes with no sign of heart activity at all, then called it.

I learned that his wife had administered CPR for about 10 minutes before the paramedics got there, but she hadn't arrived to the Emergency Department yet. I wondered why she wasn't there yet.

I soon found out. She had four children at home that she needed to get ready on Christmas morning and come to the Emergency Department. I really hate working Christmas, there is always something awful that happens.

They arrived in about 30 minutes and were placed in the family room.

I went back to talk with them. The hospital pastor grabbed my arm as I walked back. "The kids don't know he's dead; the mom knows but wants you to be the one to tell them".

I completely understood that. That information should not come from the mom, because the kids would always remember that and it would just not be a good thing psychologically for those kids.

I walked in the family room. The kids ranged in age from 8 to about 14. I sat down in front of them, their mom was to the left side in a chair.

I always start with asking what happened that morning, so they can talk about it. A girl who was 10 told me, "I went to wake daddy up for Christmas morning, but I couldn't wake him up. He looked wrong and so I screamed for mommy". The mom then told me how she did CPR and the oldest boy called 911.

"When the paramedics got there he didn't have a heartbeat or a pulse," I explained. "The paramedics tried everything to get his heart going but none of the medications would work." I explained to them that our efforts hadn't worked either, and that he had died.

The kids had already been crying when they arrived, and now everyone cried together for a few minutes. As always, I predictably had tears running down my face as well. The kids then started asking questions. The oldest daughter wanted to know if he had any pain, and I discussed no, the heart attack most likely wiped out the electrical conducting system of his heart in his sleep, and that he had no pain. One of the boys wanted to know why it happened, and I explained about the patient's coronary arteries and build-up of plaque, and that the patient had a medical history that would contribute to that. I explained that none of the kids would go home and die, kids always worry about dying in their sleep after something like this happens.

This would be horrible on any day but to have it happen on a holiday is really too much to bear for any family. We had a long talk, about 30 minutes, until they didn't have any more questions. They were a very intelligent, wonderful family, who had a horrible thing happen on Christmas Day. Their dad would be proud of them.

Consultants

In the Emergency Department, I would estimate that 75% of patients are cared for and sent home by the Emergency Physician. Sometimes their primary care providers are notified if the patient needs early follow-up, but usually the physician just receives a copy of the Emergency Department dictation of their care, along with laboratory results and x-ray reports.

In the rest of the cases however, the patient will need to be admitted and a consulting physician contacted. At the hospital where I work, we are very lucky because our attending physicians are usually very responsive and helpful, or at least don't complain too much. To be awakened at 2 in the morning, time and time again in your career, with calls from the Emergency Department, probably takes years off of our consulting physician's lives.

Often when we reach the physician, they are so tired that they barely answer our questions but mumble that they will see the patient in the morning. Most of the time that is what we want as well. The patient is stable, they just need to stay in the hospital. A good example is a patient with a hip fracture. They won't have surgery until daylight, but obviously they can't go home, and need to be admitted for IV pain medications. The orthopedist needs to be called, then he can hopefully get some sleep for a few hours before coming in.

One time, of course at 2 in the morning, I called one of my favorite pulmonologists to tell him I had a 17-year-old patient who was in severe status asthmaticus; which is asthma that will not turn around despite the typical medical therapies we give. "OK, go ahead and give him 40 mg of Inapsine and intubate him if he's not turning around with the SQ epi", he said. I paused. "With inapsine?" I asked. "Yes", he mumbled. "We are using inapsine now for status asthmaticus." He sleepily repeated how to dose it and told me he would come in. I got off the phone and stared into space for a second. I had never heard of giving Inapsine for an intubation. I didn't feel comfortable with the dose. Yet, he was a great pulmonologist whom I had known for many years.

I walked back to the patient's room. "Can you please get the Versed and Vecuronium", I said to the nurse. I just couldn't do Inapsine. I didn't even have time to read to look it up or get comfortable with it, I just couldn't do it. We went ahead and sedated and paralyzed the patient. Paralyzation is usually necessary for intubations; there are medications which specifically paralyze patients so we can get the endotracheal tube safely down their trachea. Otherwise, their muscle tone makes it difficult. We sedate them first so that they aren't aware of the feeling of being paralyzed.

About ten minutes later, my consulting pulmonologist came in. "How did the intubation go?" he asked. "Fine", I said sheepishly. "I have to tell you though, I didn't use the Inapsine. I have never used it before and I just didn't feel comfortable. I used Versed and Vecuronium".

He stared at me like I was crazy. "Why in the world would you use Inapsine for an intubation? That's for nausea!" he said, surprised.

"You told me to on the phone, remember? You said give 40 mg for intubation." I responded. He looked at me like I was crazy.

I realized that he had absolutely no memory of the conversation. He had told me to give the Inapsine, but it was in a half-awake state, and he had no recollection of it. He had managed to get himself out of bed and come in, but I don't think he ever believed me that he had told me to give Inapsine. Thank goodness I didn't listen to him even though I trusted his opinion so much.

That patient improved rapidly and went home in just several days.

On multiple occasions, I have had the physician fall asleep while I am talking to them. This has been a big problem on several occasions when I could not wake them up, even with shouting into the phone, and then we couldn't call their house back and had to keep ringing their pager or cell phone.

Some of our consultants though are remarkably helpful and thoughtful on the phone, regarding the patient's care. Recently I took care of a young gentleman from Mexico, only 22 years old. He came in with right upper abdominal pain. He had been seen in the Emergency Department two days before, for the same pain and vomiting. My partner had drawn blood work on him and it came back with elevated liver enzymes. My partner then added a hepatitis panel, which had come back positive, and he had left the patient a message so he could get follow up.

The patient came back in because he didn't completely understand the message. I discussed with the patient that he had Hepatitis B. Overall, the patient felt better, and wasn't vomiting anymore. I called our gastroenterologist to discuss the patient and to arrange follow-up.

Though I had woken the gastroenterologist at around midnight, he listened patiently to the story. He wanted to know all of the blood results. After he heard them he said, "I don't think he has acute hepatitis. I think he has probably had chronic hepatitis for a long time. I think there is something else that is going on that you are missing." The blood numbers just didn't make sense to him. After more discussion, he told me to get an ultrasound.

I ordered an ultrasound, which showed a large (14 cm) mass in the patient's liver. Further studies unfortunately demonstrated that it was liver cancer. The patient was admitted so that he could be further evaluated and get treatment. Although it was a very sad situation, it was good that the patient was diagnosed correctly and could begin treatment immediately. I appreciated that the gastroenterologist took the time to listen and think about the case.

98

Unfortunately, I have had a few true knock-down drag-outs with physicians over the years. Fortunately these have been pretty rare.

I had a chest pain patient that I strongly felt should go for immediate heart catheterization. It was a 70-year-old woman with chest pain for two hours and an abnormal EKG, though it didn't fit the exact criteria that we usually use to send a patient for heart catheterization. My concern was that she was "diaphoretic", which means sweaty, looked grey, and I really felt she was having a heart attack though the EKG didn't show it.

My phone conversation got off to a bad start with the cardiologist, when he told me "You ER docs always overread EKG's. Just put her upstairs and I'll see her in the morning." I told him he had to come into the Emergency Department, and he hung up on me. I tried to call him back, and couldn't reach him. Meanwhile, the patient was looking more distressed and her discomfort wasn't relieved with any of the medications I gave her.

I had to go see another patient, and when I came out I learned that the cardiologist had actually come in to the Emergency Department, and was sending the patient home. I went up to him, and basically we got in a huge argument which culminated with me pointing my finger in his chest and arguing my case.

After a stand-off of some sorts, he agreed to admit the patient for a workup. He did take the patient for angiogram the next day, and found she had a single lesion that needed a cardiac stent, and she did well. We did talk about it later, under calmer circumstances.

Two years ago I took care of a patient who was 35-years-old but just had to have his aortic valve repaired. He came in because he was feeling lightheaded and weak. His surgery was 7 days prior and he had gone home two days before he came back to the Emergency Department.

He was there with his wife. The nurse placed him on a monitor and already had an IV in. I reviewed his medical records, and listened to his history and examined him. He looked tired, but nothing stood out.

Suddenly, while I was talking to him, his heart rhythm changed dramatically and went into the 200's with a very narrow waveform on the monitor. It lasted literally about a minute, and by the time we had the code cart in the room it had resolved. Right at that time the echocardiogram tech arrived (an echo is like an ultrasound, but of the heart). He quickly did the echo, that showed a lot of fluid around the patient's heart, in the sac that surrounds it. This is a pericardial tamponade, and can be deadly.

I went out to call the patient's cardiothoracic surgeon, and told him my concerns. He told me some fluid around the heart is normal after surgery and that I was overreacting. I was a little surprised by his answer but told him I wanted him to come see the patient and review the echo.

Shortly after, the nurse told me that the surgeon was in the patient's room, so I walked in to listen. To my surprise, he was complaining about me to the patient and the family, and telling them that I didn't understand what an echocardiogram would look like after heart surgery. The patient's wife said, "Well, I think something is really wrong…"

Right at that time, the patient went into the rapid rhythm again. We set up to shock him but he again went out of it, back to a normal rhythm. The surgeon then reviewed the echocardiogram, told the patient he still thought I was wrong but he would take the patient back to the OR to evaluate him.

Several hours later, the surgeon did call me, which I really appreciated, to tell me that there was 800 cc of blood that had to be evacuated from around the patient's heart. Although I was kind of upset with him, I really appreciated that he came to see the patient when I asked and that he took the patient to the OR and treated the patient appropriately.

The bottom line is, different opinions exist, and when we call specialists, we are seeking their opinions. However, sometimes we don't agree with their opinions, and that creates friction. But, our responsibility is to do the right thing for the patient, and it has to be done at that exact time. I don't care how much someone yells at me or disagrees with me, as long as they do the right thing for the patient.

That is why we occasionally have "disagreements" in the Emergency Department. You can't have a meeting, you can't go to the boss, it has to be decided right then, and so friction comes with the territory. I used to stew about it for hours if I got into an argument with a consultant. Now I just consider it par for the course, and it doesn't upset me as much (as long as I get my way of course.)

A New Disease

After 20 years of practice, in 2009 we first began hearing of Swine flu in early spring. The first reports out of Mexico sounded alarming; multiple deaths were reported. The media panicked initially, there were endless videos if people wearing masks in other countries, and stories of individuals who wouldn't travel. In China and other countries individuals with fevers who were travelling were detained.

However, over summer the publicity quieted down in the media, though the infestation continued to work its way quietly around the world now.

In October, Swine flu hit with a vengeance in most of the United States. Despite six months to prepare, the vaccinations were still not available for most of the population. (Later we learned that the vaccinations were ready, but hadn't been distributed properly, and at the end of the year the unused vaccinations were all destroyed).

I have always worried about disaster preparedness in the Emergency Department since 9/11/01. While we all went through "disaster drills" before this, we considered them an administrative necessary evil, and really just went through the motions, prior to 9/11. Even before 9/11/01 though, I remember being concerned when even a four-person trauma or the winter seasonal (regular) flu would shut our Emergency Department and other Emergency Departments in our town to go on "divert" and turn away patients.

After 9/11/01, disaster planning took a new turn. Disaster planning received a huge amount of government funding; though in my observation much of the money seemed to just evaporate. We did get a nice new big tent to put up outside of the Emergency Department if we had too many patients, and a new code that was called on the overhead if there was a Mass Casualty Event, they would announce "Mass Casualty Code". That seemed somewhat funny to me; all that money that was poured into the system and that is what we got. It didn't really activate anything. What I had wanted was a system for paging all of the individuals in the hospital automatically and transport mechanisms arranged for workers to arrive in the event of a disaster, but that is still waiting.

During October, I kept hearing that Swine flu cases were on the uptick. I hadn't seen very many yet, just a trickle.

I went to work on a Friday morning and it hit, all at one time. All day long I had one flu case after another. Our hospital had not been able to procure enough vaccinations for our staff, but fortunately I had managed to get one of the rare shots the day before. Little good that will do me, I thought to myself as people coughed all over me. It takes the immunization about a week to build up your immunity.

"Code 99, room 101", I heard called overhead. This means that the Emergency Physician must leave the Emergency Department and go upstairs for a patient who is being resuscitated. I grabbed the "airway backpack" we carry and ran up.

I quickly ran up stairs and into the ICU door. As I turned into the dark hall of the ICU, I saw several people in the hall. "They can't get her tubed", one of them said to me. As I approached the crowded room, another person told me the same thing. There had been difficulty with the intubation, always a frightening situation.

I walked into the room, grabbing gloves. I quickly sized up what was happening. The pulmonologist was standing above the patient's head, attempting to intubate her. From the patient's mouth was the largest amount of frothy pink secretions I had ever seen. It looked like a volcano. I quickly grabbed the suction catheter and helped the doctor in attendance suction her, then helped position the face mask so we could ventilate her with the bag that we use.

"I can't see the cords, there are too many secretions." he said, about his prior attempts. I noticed that it was very difficult to bag air into her lungs; they seemed stiff. I asked for a Macintosh 4 blade for the intubation and a 7.0 endotracheal tube. After we got her oxygen level up, I opened her mouth, positioned my blade, and was fortunately able to see her vocal cords. I slid the tube down. Immediately, up through the tube, came a remarkable amount of pink, frothy secretions that we began to suction, but her oxygen levels slowly started to improve after she was successfully intubated.

As I spoke with the pulmonologist, I learned the patient had just given birth, and had contacted the swine flu. As we talked, I realized gratefully that a nurse had put a mask on me when I walked in the room, I hadn't even noticed it at the time. He told me about the patient's rocky course. She had given birth, and everything had gone fine. She then had mild cold symptoms, but the next day was diagnosed with pneumonia. She still looked great. That was just earlier today! By the afternoon she deteriorated and was moved into the ICU, and now was in respiratory failure and on medication to support her blood pressure.

As I walked back to the Emergency Department, this patient was on my mind. The tragedy of a young mother being so ill was devastating for everyone involved.

My first patient when I got back to the ER was a 52-day-old infant. I picked up the chart, and was walking in the room when the nurse approached me. "Look what I suctioned out of that baby", she said proudly. It was pink, frothy secretions, in a sealed plastic specimen cup. I froze.

It looked exactly like the secretions from the new mom in the ICU. I went into the room. The baby looked great, and was breast feeding, just a little fussy. I carefully examined him and talked to the parents. He had no fever, was feeding, they just brought him in because they felt he had a "cold". Normally I would have sent him home, but still reeling from the patient upstairs in the ICU, I decided to completely "wuss out" and admitted him. The pediatrician, I could tell, was unimpressed but didn't fight the admission. That was my last patient of the day.

On my way home, I felt disgusted with myself. Why did I admit that baby? I am supposed to be able to make the tough decisions. That baby looked great. He should have gone home. Instead I admitted him, probably causing financial hardship for the parents, who didn't have insurance. I had started him on Tamiflu, which isn't proven in babies, but we were all using because we were so worried about the Swine Flu at that time. There were multiple reports in the media of infants and children dying at this point who hadn't received treatment.

That night when I arrived home, I watched the news on a national TV channel about two individuals who had been seen in doctor's offices, sent home, then came back to the hospital and had died from the swine flu.

At that time, we were being told that if we took care of mild flu cases in the Emergency Department, do not offer them Tamiflu, the antiviral drug. But my feeling was, I was now scared to death of this disease; it was a new disease that seemed unpredictable; and I could not in good faith tell anyone they could not have Tamiflu if they wanted it. I would give it to my own family.

The next week, the pediatrician approached me in the hall. "Did you hear about that baby?" she asked. "He looked fine the first day, but really went downhill. He was intubated but is doing OK. His Swine culture was positive".

I thought about this for several days. Because of being "freaked out" by the patient in the ICU, the first really sick patient I'd seen with Swine flu, I had admitted the baby. No other reason than that. They both had the same pink, frothy secretions, which I had never seen before with any disease. Medicine, I thought, really is an art and not a science.

(Follow-up: After a four week ICU admission with an extremely rocky course, the young woman who had just given birth recovered and eventually went home after a rehabilitation stay. She had a complete recovery.)

Make Up

"You've got a guy with priapism for 6 hours in room 15", the nurse said as she handed me a chart.

"Interesting", I said. Priapism is when a patient gets a prolonged erection. It can occur from some medical conditions, such as sickle cell anemia. It can also occur from some medications. There are a variety of treatments we can do to stop it, such as injecting medications into the penis, although more often than not the patient has to go to the operating room for surgical intervention. If an erection goes on for too long, it can actually render a patient permanently impotent.

"He took Viagra over 6 hours ago, has had a painful erection, and is miserable," she said. I walked into the room and closed the curtain.

"Hello sir, I'm the Emergency Physician. The nurse told me about your prob…."

"Wait," he interrupted. He held his hand up to shush me. We were both quiet for a second, him looking off into space, then onto his lap covered with a sheet. I stared at him, silently.

"It went away. Right as you walked in the room. It's gone!" he said, happily.

"Maybe I should wear more makeup to work or do my hair," I offered. Both he and I got a good laugh out of it. That is the first and only time I have cured priapism by walking into a room.

Emergency Department Nurses

Emergency Department nurses truly are a breed apart. The Emergency Department is not for everyone. It is not for nurses who cannot stand on their feet on a hard floor for 12 hours and miss their bathroom and lunch breaks. It is not for nurses who mind helping vomiting patients, then running to the next bed, giving medications for a resuscitation, then in ten minutes helping hold a baby for another nurse while an IV is placed, then dealing with an out of control psychiatric patient ten minutes after that. It is not for nurses who have to have everything clean and tidy all of the time, although they do have to have everything in a certain place and God help anyone who moves it. It is not for nurses who are judgmental about social problems such as drug or alcohol addiction.

Emergency Department nurses have to be able to move rapidly from one situation to another literally within minutes. They have to deal with different staff almost every time they work, work weird hours, deal with distraught families, do tons of paperwork and charting, work one minute on a 2 day old then 5 minutes later on a 90-year-old, then either get no break or maybe a 5 minute one if they are lucky.

Emergency Department nurses have saved my butt on many occasions. I learned early to always listen to them and to trust their instincts.

The first thing you need to know is, it takes a lot to impress them. Think about an Emergency Department nurse, at the triage desk, dealing with the public as they come in all day, twelve-hour shift, day after day, for years. As they sit at the triage desk, they will be approached by say, 10-40 patients per shift, many of whom feel that their problem or their family members problem is the most important problem in the Emergency Department, which is the right and natural way for them to feel.

It can be that their child has had a sore throat for two weeks, but they want that child seen right away because tonight the child looks worse. The next patient is vomiting with the flu, routine to us, but an emergency to that patient. The next is a child with a 1 centimeter laceration on the forehead, and the parents are extremely upset. One after another, all night long.

The triage nurse has to decide who goes back first, which often drives the family members crazy if they know they were ahead, but that is how it works. Someone has to make the decision on who is the most sick, and that patient comes back first.

I will say, I don't know how they do triage. It would drive me crazy to sit out there. Yet they do a remarkably good job at it. They know that that patient over there, the pale man who checked in with pain in his upper abdomen pain and who doesn't complain about waiting, may be actually having a heart attack. They know that the 21-year-old girl who has a stomach ache probably has appendicitis by the way she walks, and is getting the next bed back, no matter how much the woman with chronic back pain and 20 prior Emergency Department visits complains about her wait. These are the type of decisions the Emergency Department nurse must make. And they must make those decisions based on being able to spend only a few minutes listening to and examining a patient who they have never met before.

We have one nurse, Sheila, who has worked in the Emergency Department literally forever. She is from the South, is about 50 now, but still a true beauty. She is tall, with blond hair, and of course that great Southern accent. She never gets rattled, never gets upset. And I know if she tells me to get in a room to see a patient right away that I had better get moving.

One time she brought a patient back from triage, a 44-year-old woman. "Mary, can you go take a look at her? I think she looks a little grey," she said calmly. I went in immediately. The woman was thin, and very anxious. She told me about some chest discomfort she was having. "I'm under a lot of stress, I have a new boss," she said. She told me more about her work situation. She did tell me she smoked ½ pack per day as well. I ordered an EKG which was stone-cold normal. I went ahead and ordered blood work.

"Well Sheila," I said to the nurse, "normal EKG, I don't know. We'll get a troponin." Sheila said, "There's just something about her that makes me nervous." I thought about this, as not much of anything made Sheila nervous. But my thoughts were interrupted by the impending arrival of a Code 3 ambulance, with a patient who had lost his pulse and blood pressure.

While running the code, Sheila came in the room. "That patient is having chest pain again", she said. "Who?" I responded, distractedly, as I was involved with this new patient. "The one in room 12, the 44-year-old woman.". "Well, I won't be in for a bit. Her EKG was completely normal, we're just waiting on blood work." Then I thought about Sheila and her sixth sense, and also the fact that she was interrupting me during a code, which she would not do unless she was really concerned. "Can you get another EKG?" I asked. Within a couple of minutes, Sheila appeared, EKG in hand. Sure enough, it showed that the patient was having an anterior myocardial infarction (heart attack). Once again, Sheila was right on. The patient went immediately to the cath lab for angioplasty and did fine.

I have probably 20 more similar situations with this one nurse. It is almost to the point that if she tells me to come in the room, I grab the resuscitation equipment. And I have similar stories with many of our other nurses.

But, she does know how to separate the wheat from the chaff. She does not abide drama well, and has no patience at all for patients who should not be in the Emergency Department at all. And she knows who should be and shouldn't be, trust me.

One time she got back from a lovely Mexico vacation with her husband. She had been gone for two weeks, and came back tan and rested looking. "I'm actually in a good mood," she volunteered. "I actually feel like helping people again." "Yeah, it is amazing what a vacation can do," I said in passing.

Shortly after that, she came back from triage. "Well, I timed myself to see how long I could go after my vacation without rolling my eyes while I was at triage." She paused. " Seven minutes," she said. "What happened?" I laughed. "Your next patient has a pool ball in his rectum. He says he fell on it".

Well, I have to say, I would roll my eyes too. At least she does it when she turns around, not in front of the patient, which is all I can ask for.

Even though she is often very jaded and cynical, I once saw this same nurse spend two hours cleaning up a 65-year-old woman who lived on a farm. The woman was working in a muddy barnyard, when she suffered a major stroke. She was paralyzed on one side. She laid in the muck and manure for over 8 hours, in the rain, before someone found her. She came in completely caked, with the mud and manure all over her skin. We had to rush her to CT first, then Sheila sat with her, gently talking to her and sponging her with a wet wash cloth, until she was clean and had at least some of her dignity back. I do know if that was me, I would want a nurse like Sheila.

But fess up about the foreign body if she is taking care of you. She knows you didn't fall on it.

Differences of Opinion

"Headache", the chart listed as a chief complaint of my next patient coming back. I saw them walk the patient back to the room, a woman age approximately 50. She walked normally and appeared well. I went in to talk with her.

"I feel dizzy, and I've had a headache for two days", she said. She had no history of headaches. She worked as a nurse in our hospital. When I examined her she was somewhat tender on her left neck, on the back of the neck. Probably muscle pain, but worst case scenario, I wonder if she could have a dissection of her vertebral artery in her neck, a very rare cause of headache. I discussed this with her. I told her I would order a CT scan with angiogram of her head and neck to look at the arteries.

"Actually, I would rather have an MRI if that is OK. I talked with my coworker and that is what she thought I should have", she said. "Well, that is reasonable", I said. It would show the same things. After more discussion, I ordered an MRI/MRA of the brain and neck which would also show the arteries. Very often, health care providers have very specific requests when they are seen medically.

This takes several hours to perform, so I continued on seeing other patients. Finally I got the call that the MRI/MRA was completely normal. I spoke with the relieved patient and sent her home.

The next day, while signing off on charts, I called her at home. "I still have a headache, and I'm still dizzy", she said. I was worried about her, so I asked her to return. I was off shift, so I told her my partner would see her.

I read her chart the next day. She had come in and got a CT/CTA this time, and it was completely normal.

The next day I worked, and I called her again. Her son answered. "She is really sick", he said, "she's in bed". I asked to speak with her. Her headache was worse. I told her she had better come back in, thinking possibly we should have obtained a lumbar puncture to rule out infection or small bleed. She didn't want to come back but agreed.

After she arrived, we started an IV and gave her pain medication. I called my favorite radiologist, "Jim, I just don't know what to do next. I'll probably do a lumbar puncture. We did both an MRI and a CT on this lady, would you mind just looking at them again before I do an LP?" I asked.

He pulled up the films on his computer. "Oh, do you mean this lady who has a vertebral dissection on the left?"

"What?!" I asked, completely shocked. Both of her films had been read out by excellent radiolologists as completely normal. But another set of eyes looking at it found an obvious abnormality that could have led to stroke for this patient.

The patient was admitted to the ICU and received Heparin, the treatment in this situation. She did well and was discharged. But it did prove my long-time theory, that medical tests are medical tests, nothing more nothing less, and that the only real answers are in talking with the patient and to keep looking for answers. And sometimes get just one more opinion from someone who is really smart.

Threesome

The heavy double doors of the Emergency Department swung open and I quickly walked through, wanting to get coffee before my shift started. I walked thru the hallway and looked over to the patient care area. One of my partners, McBee, was sitting at the end of the bed on a stool. The patient had her legs up with a large amount of blood on the sheets on the end of the bed.

I was appalled. I assumed it was a miscarriage, and he was performing a pelvic examination. He hadn't shut the curtain? I couldn't believe that. I made a turn and walked over to close the curtain.

As I approached, McBee looked over at me, and as he turned his head I could see the patient was a man. I quickly closed the curtain and went for my coffee, quite confused.

After changing into scrubs and with coffee in hand, I returned to the desk as my shift started.

I heard McBee now calling for blood products, and saw the nurses scurrying around. The secretary then told me what happened.

The patient was working at a dance, when he met an attractive woman. He hit it up with her and invited her back to his place. She asked if she could bring a friend. The patient thought he was in heaven. Needless to say, alcohol was involved in large quantities.

The three went to his apartment where he promptly undressed. They saw that he was uncircumcised, and for some unknown reason were "grossed out", in his words. They didn't want to have sex with an uncircumcised man.

Taking matters into his own hands, literally, he took a razor blade and got in a bathtub.

He proceeded to try to circumcise himself, but in the process lopped off the bottom 1/3 of his penis.

When the women saw the bloody mess, they somehow thought he had been attacked, and called 911 for police. Police arrived and cordoned off the scene. They then realized what had happened after somewhat of a delay, and called paramedics.

Ultimately, the patient was taken to the operating room after receiving two units of blood and underwent surgical repair of what was left of his penis.

The Power of Positive Thinking

One of my dear friends called me, an old Emergency doc at the coast. "I'm sending you an 80-year-old male, I think he's got an abdominal aneurysm," he said. An aneurysm is an enlargement of an artery, in this case the biggest artery that goes down through the abdomen. These can become so large that they rupture, and are often fatal.

The doc had been working at the coast forever. I knew him from when I was a resident and used to moonlight at his hospital. It is a small hospital that sees every complaint, from minor complaints to major trauma. If a patient has a major problem they need to be transferred to a tertiary care hospital.

It took two hours, but the patient arrived by ambulance. They could not fly him because the coast was fogged in.

Despite the fact that the coast hospital at that time had no CT scanner at night, I suspected when I examined the elderly man that the diagnosis was correct. I ordered a stat CT scan, and blood work including type and cross. The gentleman was by himself, so I asked him for his wife's phone number.

"Oh, don't call her now. I don't want to upset her," he said calmly.

"Does she know you came here from the coast?" I asked.

"No, I didn't want them to tell her. It is the middle of the night and I don't want to wake her up, she isn't a good sleeper," he answered.

Against my judgment, I let it go at this time and he went off to CT scan, which showed a very large, greater than 10 centimeter, aneurysm with possible small leak. This is very often a fatal diagnosis. If an aneurysm is found on a patient before it causes pain or bleeding, it can often be repaired electively and the patient will do well. However, once there are signs of rupture, mortality can be as high as 90%.

I called the vascular surgeon and the operating room. I went back in the room to talk with the patient. "OK, I'm going to call your wife now, so can you please give me her number?" I asked after I explained the situation to him.

"No, just let her sleep," he said. "I'll call her in the morning." I didn't want to scare him, but I told him that this was extremely serious and that there was a chance he could die from it, and I felt we had to notify her. He was very sweet, but would not let me call. I basically talked myself blue in the face at this point, but he would not give me permission to call his wife.

He took my hand in his, and said sweetly, "Everything will be fine. Don't you worry."

At this point, I gave up as the OR team was there. They wheeled him and his 90% mortality risk off for emergency surgery.

The next day, I called the ICU and spoke with the nurse. "He's doing great!" she said, surprised. "He is already wide awake, off the ventilator, and talking up a storm". His wife had arrived that morning, after her peaceful night sleep.

Although I still feel bad about not notifying her, as I would want to be notified in that situation, I thought maybe his thinking that everything would be fine actually affected his outcome. There are some things we just do not know.

Advanced Directive

"Code 3 ambulance coming in," said the charge nurse. "Suicide attempt."

Taking care of patients who have attempted suicide is a very frequent event in the Emergency Department. The vast majority are a "cry for help", often a young individual, most often a woman (studies bear this out), who has taken several of some type of medication after becoming upset by something, or makes some cutting marks on themselves.

In many cases, we can arrange counseling in the Emergency Department, observe the patient, and when they feel safe and have a family member to go home with we will discharge them for psychiatric follow-up. I would estimate that I see a patient with this situation once or twice per shift.

Some are far more serious, where a patient takes a very large amount of medication or attempts something equally as fatal. These patients are typically evaluated, cleared medically, and then admitted to the hospital for psychiatric care. What is always surprising to me is how often these patients call for help themselves. They take the overdose or inflict harm of some type on themselves, and then call 911 or a family member to come get them. It shows how much they really want and need help.

When the ambulance pulled up, they arrived with a very ill—appearing female, who they had brought from a hotel. "She checked in yesterday," the paramedic reported. "The maid tried to get in today, and they found her like this," he said.

The paramedics had already placed an IV and had her on oxygen, but she was clearly in respiratory distress and needed intubating. "She left a note," he handed it to our nurse.

We resuscitated the patient. After she was stabilized, I read the note while I was still in the room. She addressed it to a member of her family, and first she apologized to them. It said she couldn't deal with her diagnosis anymore, and couldn't take the pain, so she had decided to do this. She talked about where she wanted her possessions and her pet to go.

I went out and looked her up in the computer. She had a diagnosis of Lymphoma, and although she wasn't end-stage, she was under aggressive treatment. She was on pain medications. Her husband had left her two years before.

She was a retired nurse. She probably didn't want her family to find her at home, so she had checked into a hotel. She put on a nightgown, and put plastic sheeting on the bed underneath her. Classic nurse, she didn't want to make anyone clean up after the mess she knew she would make after she overdosed. Then, she took the near-fatal overdose and laid down on the plastic sheeting. This patient did not want to be found alive. She wanted to finish the job she had started.

The law is, we have to resuscitate these patients. There is such a thing as a Physician Assisted Suicide for terminal patients in our state, but they have to go through a length evaluation process before that is approved. If someone tries to kill themselves on their own, the paramedics and health care personnel have to resuscitate them if 911 is called.

I remember a time when I was judgmental about patients who attempted suicide, even if it was just a gesture. Now, after 20 years of seeing various situations, I have learned that there are patients who are having so much pain that it seems like the only option, though most people would not agree with this. The patient's feel that other people's lives will be better if they are gone. They can't get out of the dark hole that they are in.

This lady was sent to the ICU, where she woke up, had psychiatric counseling, and was discharged. I never heard what happened to her after that. I do not know if she had any happiness in the rest of her life, but I do think about her and the only feeling I have is empathy, and the wish that I could do something to help her.

Over the years, I've developed my own theory that patients chose their type of suicide attempt based on what they are feeling inside. Overdose patients feel like they are being poisoned inside by their thoughts and emotions, jumpers have so much inner pain that they want to get rid of it by causing physical pain, those who hang themselves feel in their regular life like they are being strangled. That is just my theory, because I spend a lot of time thinking about these patients.

We usually never know what happens to these patients after they leave our Emergency Department, or what the rest of their lives are like.

During this recession we have had more and more suicide attempts as people have become more desperate and lose hope. The Medical Examiner in our county told me this year on Christmas Day that he had gone to five completed suicides at people's homes, a tragic sign of the times.

Complaints

We all get them, no matter how hard you try. Someone will not be happy and will complain to the hospital administration. You may or may not feel they are justified, but complaints will come.

I took care of 50-year-old patient who came in with right pelvic pain. I examined her and took a detailed history. I ordered blood work, a urine test, and an ultrasound. All were completely normal. I re-examined her, she was still quite painful. I told her I was very concerned and ordered a CT scan to rule out appendicitis, though her story wasn't consistent with appendicitis, no vomiting, no fever, no elevated white blood cell count, and the pain was lower than her appendix. The CT was completely normal.

I re-examined her again. She was even more painful. I told her the tests were all normal but I thought we should admit her for ob-servation. I consulted both a surgeon and gynecologist, and she was admitted. Her pain was slightly better with the pain medications we had given her.

Two months later, I received a complaint through our director about her. She had written a letter, saying I hadn't diagnosed her. I reviewed her records. After admission, both the gynecologist and sur-geon saw her, but her tests continued normal. A repeat ultrasound and repeat CT were normal. On the fourth day, a third ultrasound was obtained, that showed a possible abscess in the right fallopian tube, very rare for a patient in this age group. She was taken to the OR and received IV antibiotics and it cleared up.

At first I was indignant. I had done all the tests and they were normal, and it took four days for a test to be abnormal, even with two specialists looking at her. But, from her point of view, I hadn't made the diagnosis, she had a long hospital course, and she thought I should have diagnosed her in the Emergency Department.

Another complaint I had I didn't take quite as seriously. I was called up to the main hospital floor for a Code Blue. I was directed into the men's bathroom, next to the cafeteria. I ran thru the door and saw several people gathered around near the stall.

There, lying face down, was a male about age 30. We rolled him over and he was completely blue in color. He also had a needle and syringe in his arm, he had been injecting Heroin and had gone into respiratory arrest from it. We cut off his shift. He had a pulse. We bagged him with an Ambu bag, then intubated him, and he rapidly improved. We then took him to the Emergency Department.

Once there, he was wide awake, and pulled out his endotracheal tube and IV. He started screaming that he wanted to leave. I had a discussion with him that he should stay for an evaluation but he refused, and I could not legally keep him there. He stormed out of the Emergency Department, then actually went immediately up to Quality Management where he demanded that we pay for the shirt we had cut off of him during the resuscitation.

I found out later that he had been visiting his girlfriend who was in the ICU for a heroin overdose. It is the only time I have had a Code Blue sign out Against Medical Advice. And we didn't pay for the shirt.

Recently I had a dad bring in his four year old for a one centimeter face laceration. He had taken the child first to his own doctor, who told him the child should have a plastic surgeon. This is not an uncommon occurrence. I feel completely comfortable taking care of this child's laceration, but the dad now feels he must have a plastic surgeon. That is definitely his right. I told him I would contact the plastic surgeon immediately.

I placed the call, and of course the plastic surgeon was in surgery. I went back and told the dad that the surgeon would come but that it would take an hour. We would start the child on antibiotics and wash his wound while we waited though. "Well, then call another plastic surgeon", he said. "Sir, we only have one plastic surgeon on call, and it is Friday night at 7, so I felt lucky that she will be able to come in especially as she is in the operating room". "Well, how would you repair it?" he asked. He obviously didn't want to wait. I explained to him the approach I would use. "That isn't what my doctor said should be done. I want to wait for the plastic surgeon". "That is no problem", I said, and asked the technician to set up a suture tray for the plastic surgeon.

In the meantime, we got a critically ill child in the room right next to that dad, and there is no way he could not have heard the resuscitation going on with this 2-year-old. The resuscitation took almost an hour. When I came out, a nurse approached me. She said that dad was so angry that he wasn't getting updates on when the plastic surgeon would come that he left for another hospital. "Wow, I think that will be tough for that kid", I said. "They will probably have an even longer wait". Right then the plastic surgeon arrived. I told him the father had left and he was very upset, venting on us.

"Also, the father said he's going to file a complaint against you", the nurse informed me.

All I could do was take it in stride, and go back and do my charting. You just aren't going to make everyone happy, no matter how much you try. There are many people who work with the public who will understand this, but it still doesn't make you feel good, especially when you feel like you are trying to do your best for every patient.

I have made my share of mistakes over the years. One of my partners calls Emergency Medicine "the art of making urgent decisions with inadequate information". I often think of that quote because it is so true.

While it sounds easy to say you should never be judgmental, the fact is, you have to be, all of the time. From the second you meet a patient you are listening to them, thinking about their responses, thinking about what is the worst thing they could have. That is the tenant of Emergency Medicine: You have to always think, "What is the worst thing that I could miss in this patient?" Needless to say, that definitely leads to over-ordering of tests.

I used to worry about over-ordering and over-spending, but eventually I decided it was the least of my worries. The biggest worry would be having something bad happen to a patient because I didn't do a test.

My line of thinking, which others may disagree with, is that if a patient has presented to the Emergency Department, their issue must be treated as an Emergency. Now, to be completely honest, I would estimate that only 20% of patients seen in the Emergency Department really need to be seen there, but you have to give everyone the benefit of the doubt. For one thing, you don't know them, you don't know their pain tolerance, and you can't think that you do even for one second. Also, sometimes people just get scared, and need to be reassured that they are OK, and that is part of why we are there, and why we have jobs.

However, despite my best intentions, I have had some misses over the years and I would be lying if I said I didn't.

When I had been in practice for about 5 years, I took care of a delightful 50-year-old man who was the head of an important company in our area. He came in with a headache. "You know, I just never get headaches, but my mother died of an aneurysm so I thought I should get it checked out." His headache had started over the last 3 days, and was on the left side. His examination was completely normal.

I did a CT scan (in those days we didn't have CTs that were done with dye to show the arteries, called CT angiograms), and it was completely normal. Because I was still worried about him, I did a lumbar puncture to rule out a very small subarachnoid bleed that wouldn't show up on CT. The fluid was sent to the lab and tested completely normal.

I discussed the normal findings with him. He was very relieved, and felt better with the medications we had given him. I spoke with his physician so he could get follow-up.

The next day I called him at home and he was still having pain. I wasn't at work but urged him to go back in. My partner did an MRI of his head, and it was normal.

The day after that, the patient went to his regular doctor, who sent him to a vascular surgeon. The vascular surgeon fortunately did an angiogram (not a CT angiogram like we have now, back then we actually had to take the patient to the cath lab and inject dye into their arteries, kind of a big procedure) which showed an aneurysm that hadn't shown up on either test!

Fortunately, he did well. I still think about this though, because it could have been a complete disaster. I had felt that I had thoroughly worked him up, but he still had something that we missed.

Another more recent miss leaves me shaking my head, and makes me think, to be honest, that my job is really hard.

I took care of a very pleasant 75-year-old woman. She had multiple medical problems including diabetes, past heart attack, kidney disease, and sleep apnea. She weighed over 350 pounds. She was in now for 3 days of diarrhea. She wasn't vomiting and had no fever. I checked blood tests on her, her electrolytes and a CBC which were normal. For no great scientific reason I did an EKG; mainly because she looked generally so unhealthy, not for any real medical reason, and it was normal. Part of my thinking was, right or wrong, this lady could come in any given day with heart disease. She had no diarrhea in the

Emergency Department and couldn't give us a sample. She felt better and could eat and drink and walk around with no problems.

The next day, I learned she had returned. She had gone home, and the next morning felt poorly, and had returned. Her EKG was unchanged but her blood tests showed she had a small heart attack (non ST elevation Myocardial Infarction)! This really bothered me. Granted, with her health problems and morbid obesity, she could have a heart attack any day, and there were no indications for admission at all when I saw her, but it just really drove home to me that sometimes you just aren't going to see everything coming. Fortunately, she did well, after a prolonged hospital stay. I was glad though that I had done the EKG the prior day and that it was normal.

I can truly tell you, there is no worse feeling then when you feel you've missed something with a patient. It is a devastating feeling that lasts for a long time.

One night when I was working with one of my new partners, he was telling me about an elderly patient he had sent home with abdominal pain, and he was worried about him. He had done a laboratory workup and x-rays, which were normal, and the patient looked well overall. While we talked about it, he pulled up the x-rays and we re-looked at them.

As he looked at them for his second time, he said "Is that a little calcium on his aorta on the lateral? It looks a little big…" "You now, you maybe be right", I said, peering at it very closely. "I missed an aortic aneurysm!" he said, visibly upset. Sometimes in the elderly, when the aorta enlarges, the edges are calcified, and you can see the enlarged outline on a plain x-ray. It can be subtle and easy to miss. It was now about 2 in the morning and he had sent the patient home several hours prior.

He went and got the patient's phone number and started calling, but no answer. He tried other relative's numbers that were listed on the chart with no luck. My partner was distraught and frantic, and angry at himself. He kept desperately redialing the same numbers.

I got busy and didn't know what was going on with the situation for awhile, then I heard from the charge nurse that the patient was back in the Emergency Department, and that the surgeon was arriving to take him for repair of his aneurysm.

I saw my young partner. "How did you get a hold of him?" I asked.

"I called the Highway Patrol and they went to his house and woke him up and drove him here!" he said, relieved. I started laughing.

Now that was service. I also credited my partner. Not everyone would go to such extreme measures to problem solve, and he had really gone the extra yard, which no doubt saved the patient's life. Of course, the situation and the stress probably took ten years off my partner's life.

Language Barrier

"Sore throat", the chart said as the Chief Complaint. I looked at the age of the patient. It was a 9 month old boy. I wondered to myself how the parents knew he had a sore throat at that age. Interesting.

I walked in the room. The family were immigrants from Vietnam, and spoke very little English. I asked the nurse to page the interpreter to come in. It was 10 at night, this could take hours.

Now, we have phone interpreter services, which are great. We can call any time, day or night, and get an interpreter immediately over a speaker phone in any language. But until about 2005 at our hospital, we had to find an interpreter , and they had to drive to the hospital. This was easy if it was a common language like Spanish, but once you go into more rare languages or even rarer dialects, it could take hours.

I continued to try to talk with the family. At least I could examine the baby without the interpreter. "My baby has a bone in his throat," the mother said. OK, what does that mean? He has a vertebrae that they think is hurt? Are they saying something else that I don't understand?

"A bone?" I asked.

"Yes, yes!" everyone in the room agreed, nodding their heads, happy that I was figuring it out. I examined the child's mouth carefully. The throat looked completely normal.

I shook my head, "It looks OK,", I said to them, hopefully.

"No, no, not OK. Bone in his throat," the mother explained again, very politely. "Bone in his throat", the rest of the room repeated, nodding.

After my examination, I exited the room. The secretary told me the translator service was having difficulty finding an interpreter, it could be hours. Great.

"Well, let's go try and take a really good look, or I guess I could do an x-ray," I said to the nurse. She went in with me, and sat in a chair on the room. She took the child, and held him on her lap with one arm around his chest and another gently holding his head, very slightly arching his head back. I took another tongue depressor.

I gave his tongue a good gag, and there it was: A fish bone, lodged right in his tonsil. I couldn't see it without gagging him. "Oh, it's a bone!" I said brilliantly. "Yes, yes a bone!" the family all agreed with the idiot doctor. They had only told me this ten times by now.

I had the tech bring me a forceps, and with one more gagging with the tongue depressor, was able to remove it. The family all clapped their hands, delighted. The baby immediately began drinking from his bottle. What I finally found out is that the baby had grabbed a small bit of fish off someone's plate at dinner, and it had a bone in it.

I am always amazed when I take care of families that come here from other countries. I can't imagine being dropped in another country with my child, and trying to navigate the housing situation, travel, jobs, and healthcare. Currently I have tried to learn Spanish for years, and still struggle with it.

The happy, polite family thanked me and the nurse about 100 times as they left. I know it sounds corny, but these are exactly the situations that made me go into Emergency Medicine. Something fixable, being able to help with some small situation for a family like this, it really is a privilege.

"Fatigue"

Whenever I see "fatigue" as a chief complaint on a chart, I have to say that my cynicism gets the best of me. As a person who works night shifts, I rarely feel that the patients who complain of fatigue are as tired as I often am after I have worked a few night shifts.

I was in the middle of a very busy shift when a chart came up with "fatigue" as a chief complaint. The patient was a 72-year-old female. Great. Huge workup, no answers. Here we go again.

I went to see the patient. She was a very delightful woman, accompanied by two friends. She volunteered at another hospital in town, and she "just felt so tired". I could really get no specifics out of her. She had volunteered that day and just felt wiped out. No fever, no chest pain, no shortness of breath, nothing.

Her friends were very concerned about her. "She is never like this", they said. But again, they couldn't be very specific. She didn't look pale to them, she hadn't complained of anything.

She had volunteered at the same hospital six days a week for over 15 years. It was a hospital where I did my residency, a big University hospital.

I ordered the usual, laboratory work, EKG, urine test. All were normal. I did a blood test that the heart releases if it is having damage, called the troponin, also normal.

I went back in to talk to her and to discharge her. We started chatting about the hospital where she volunteered and where I used to work. I had recently been there to visit a friend's son. "Boy, it sure has spread out now, with all those new buildings," I said. We talked about all of the new departments there, and how much it had grown.

"That's the thing I noticed," she said. "Usually I walk 3-4 miles a day there. I wear a pedometer. But today, I walked down just one hall and couldn't walk anymore."

I looked at her for a minute. This was a lady who had never been in the Emergency Department, who volunteered everyday, who now had this complaint. I decided just to admit her. What a sieve I am, I thought to myself.

Two days later I pulled up her records. Her doctor, a very good internist, did a type of a chemical stress test, which was very abnormal, and she ended up having a completely abnormal angiogram that lead to a 5 vessel heart bypass surgery. Amazing.

I don't know what lesson to take out of this, but this happens all of the time. You will see 1,000 patients with the same complaint and find nothing, then with one patient, they will have something very abnormal where if you had sent them home they might have had a fatal outcome. It really is frightening sometimes to think about it, and it also makes me wish I could have more time with each patient. If we hadn't had that little conversation about how she tired out in a long hallway, her diagnosis could have been delayed or missed completely.

Animals

When I grew up, we had a neighbor who took his beautiful Great Dane for a walk on a snowy, icy night after dark. As he walked down the street, he slipped on the ice and fell, fracturing his femur. The dog thought he was playing, grabbed the hat off my neighbor's head, and ran off.

My neighbor described later how he lay there after the fall in pain, not being able to move, and thinking things couldn't get worse, until he realized that now he was laying there without a hat. Finally another neighbor driving home saw him.

I often think of that story now, because of the amount of "animal-related" injuries we see at work. We all love our pets, but I can't lie, there are an amazing amount of injuries related to them. Of course there are the dog bites, often happening with what are always described as the nicest dogs, but even the nicest dog does not appreciate a 5-year-old taking his toy or bone.

The most common thing I see though is people tripping over their pets when they are carrying objects. This is an unending source of patients in the Emergency Department. My own dog, Amy, sleeps on the exact middle step of our stairs so she can see what is going on, and we have tripped over her many times.

I had a boy who was 8 or 9 come in with a dog bite, accompanied by his mother. I introduced myself and asked about the injury, then briefly examined him. He had a large dog bite on his left cheek, unfortunately it would need stitches. We don't like to stitch dog bites unless we have to, because of the risk of infection. But if the wound is in a cosmetically important area, our hand is forced.

His mother was Vietnamese, but spoke some English. She was very skinny and seemed nervous. In the room with them was another older woman who seemed upset. I couldn't figure out the dynamics in the room at all.

I told them I would come back when the suture tray was upset, and went off to check on other patients. When I was walking down the hall a short time later, the boy's mother was in the back hall. She pulled me aside, and told me the dog had bit the boy before, on the arm and on the stomach. She was very secretive and guarded about it, and spoke in whispers. I was thoroughly confused. There was something really wrong I could tell, but I couldn't figure out what.

When I started the boy's laceration, now that he had pain medications and was numbed, I realized that it was a much more extensive wound then I initially thought. It took quite awhile to take care of it. The whole time I was in there, I re-assured and talked with him, but mom and the other woman sat silently. I started asking questions about the dog.

The older woman snapped at me suddenly. "I've told him to leave that dog alone!" She said. I asked what kind of dog it was and she said it was Rottweiler. "He is supposed to leave it alone, and he is always going near it". I decided not to say anything at this time, because I now noticed mom was sitting with her head bowed and eyes down. There was some situation here that just wasn't clear to me, but I knew there was something not OK for this kid to go back to.

After I was done, I told them that I would have to report this as a dog bite, and since the dog had bitten the kid before they needed to get rid of it.

The older lady now yelled at me. "It's his fault, not the dogs!" she said angrily. "He keeps provoking it!" While kids definitely can provoke dogs, the fact that this kid now had been bitten several times put him at risk.

"Well, you need to get rid of it," I said, "And I'm going to send someone out to check to be sure you do".

After my shift I spent 30 minutes on the phone with a deputy, trying to get him to go to the house. "Do you think the kid is in immediate danger?" He asked me. "Well, he could be", I said. "Look", he said, "there is nothing I can do here. If they want to own a dog, it is their choice, I can't take away their dog." I asked for his supervisor but he said he was unavailable. After talking myself blue in the face to him, I gave up for the night.

The next morning, I called the County Police back but this time asked for the Chief. I was told he was in a meeting so I asked that they get him out. After 5 minutes on hold, he came to the phone and I explained my concern, and that the officer said they could do nothing about it. He listened carefully, then said, "You were told the wrong information. That dog absolutely needs to be removed, and I will call you as soon as I have resolution to this."

Several hours later, he called and told me that an officer went out there. There were multiple Vietnamese women in the house with small children, the older woman, and 5 Rottweiler's. He also did not understand what was going on, but talked the owner, the older woman, into relinquishing the Rottweiler. They were going to try to find out more about what was going on at the house, but I never heard follow-up. I felt really bad for that mom though, and hoped things worked out for her. I had a feeling she didn't have many choices in her life but knew she had to get out of there somehow.

I am a big animal lover. But in situations like this we have to intervene, but I just end up feeling like there was no happy ending for anyone. The child's safety though has to be the first concern.

Occasionally we have people who actually bring animals into the Emergency Department.

I went to take care of a 13-year-old. The chart read "bit by a mouse". Patients worry about mice because they are concerned about rabies so they come in to the Emergency Department. However, mice bites actually aren't concerning for rabies because rodents don't carry rabies, but it would be a concern for infection. I walked in the room reading the nurse's notes as I went. I spoke as I walked, "I hear you got bitten by a mouse?" but as I looked up I involuntarily screamed. The dad was standing there, holding a dead mouse by the tail. I backed up and slammed the door I am ashamed to say.

I sought out our tech, Ralph, who is the most wonderful person in the world in many ways, and has worked in our Emergency Department for 20 years. I explained what happened, and he bravely ventured into the room and got the offending mouse in a plastic bag. Unfortunately the bag was clear, and everyone could see the mouse, traumatizing more of our staff until it was disposed of.

The dad had brought in the mouse thinking it should be tested for rabies, completely understandable. I apologized to them both for my reaction and took care of the bite wound.

Another time, in the middle of the night, a chart came up that said "snake bite". For some reason the details of the case completely escape me, but I know it was the patient's own pet snake. The word came back from the triage nurse that the patient had brought in the snake.

Our secretary, Betty, immediately panicked. She had a deathly phobia of snakes. "They had better not bring that thing back here", she said, actually she said that multiple times. I assured her I would go right in the room and check. I am not as afraid of snakes as I am of mice.

I went in the room, and learned that the triage nurse had already disposed of the snake, which the patient had killed prior to arrival. While I was in the room though, I suddenly heard loud screaming coming from the central desk area. I thought there must be an assault or a violent psychiatric patient, so I ran out of the room. Betty was half standing/half kneeling on the chair and counter, completely hysterical and could not be calmed down. She screamed over and over.

What had happened, is that one of our male techs, knowing Betty's fear, had put plastic tubing in a white plastic bag, then walked up to her and said, "Oh, here's the snake, they want it sent to the lab", and threw it on the desk. She completely freaked out, and could not be calmed down.

She actually had to leave her shift and go home, as she could not function after that. That was a prank that really back-fired I might add as now we had no secretary for the rest of the night.

I took care of a lovely elderly woman last summer who came in after she started feeling short of breath, worsening over several days. She had driven herself in. I told her I wanted to do a chest x-ray and blood work.

"Well, I will get the tests if you want, but do you think it's too hot in the car for my little dogs?" she asked. She had two poodles in the car she said. She had hoped she would just be in and out of the Emergency Department, and had left her windows cracked and parked undercover, but was very worried about them. It was fairly hot outside, so I asked our security guard if he could go get them out, which he gladly did.

Next time I walked by her room, there were two little gray poodles, running around the room. They were so cute. I went in and talked with her; she had gotten both of them from the Humane Society when there former owner died. Everyone in the department was so happy to see them, and she had every nurse and tech in the department in the room petting them while she was there.

We ended up having to admit her, and a friend was going to come get the dogs. They wheeled her upstairs, with the dogs lying next to her happily on the stretcher.

We did have one lady who kept bringing her "service dog", a huge, mangy mixed-breed with long, wiry hair, who had absolutely no manners. I was very suspicious that this dog was actually a service dog as it seemed poorly trained and would lift its leg on the stretcher wheels or garbage can in the room, unleashing a gallon of urine. It was amazing. But if a patient says it is a service dog we have to believe them. And it did have the vest on.

The patient would occasionally have to be admitted, and for reasons I won't go into there were some difficulties in caring for her. One of my favorite internists, when I called him that she was in the Emergency Department, told me that he would have to call his partner. He had been relieved from the case because the dog had bitten him the last time she had been admitted. I told him he sounded awfully happy about that. After I would admit her, I would hear complaints for days about the nurses having to take it outside, or worse, when they had "carpet emergencies" upstairs. The dog must have weighed 100 pounds so it couldn't have been fun.

Anyway, I can't really make fun of others and their pets too much. When my father was admitted to the hospital for his third back surgery at age 75, and became quite ill, I smuggled up his little 5 pound dog to visit him. I had to carry it up 7 flights of stairs so no one would see me. Pets do make a huge difference in our lives.

Teaching Cases

Part of practicing medicine is teaching others who follow in your footsteps. It is an integral part of medicine to pass on knowledge to the next generation. That said, in the Emergency Department I typically don't like working with residents and medical students. Nothing personal at all, I just like to focus on each patient without being interrupted, and our department is so busy it is one extra thing going on.

But at our hospital we have residents, and I try to follow the rules and hopefully pass something on to them when possible. We need to allow them to participate and I realize it is a vital function.

On a night shift, near the end of my shift, I was called up for an intubation in the ICU. When there is a code or an emergent airway issue upstairs we are called up. If the "code team" is there, which includes a house-staff resident, we are supposed to let them run the code unless they need help, and they can attempt an airway but if they can't get it then we take over. Oral intubation is a procedure that we do more often in the Emergency Department so it is something that we can often help with in difficult situations.

When I arrived, the patient had a blood pressure and pulse but was in respiratory failure from pneumonia. She was a thin 65-year-old woman. The resident was trying to intubate with the Glidescope, a lighted device that lets you see the trachea on a screen.

The resident attempted to pass the tube. "Are you in?" I asked. "Yes, I'm pretty sure" he answered. I see some fluid in the tube, listen to the patient's chest with my stethoscope, it doesn't sound like good air movement, then I look back at the tube and see more clear fluid.

"Is that stomach contents?" I ask. I immediately start pulling the tube and we assist the patient's ventilation with an Ambu bag. As soon as the oxygen level is up the resident wanted to try again. I usually let them twice if it is a fairly stable patient. He attempts again with the Glidescope, and immediately the patient starts vomiting a large amount of clear fluid. It is coming out like from an open conduit, just frothing out of her.

I grab a larnygoscope, Mac 4, my favorite, and take a look. To my surprise the patient has very narrow mouth opening and what we call an "anterior" airway, I can't see her cords at all. On top of it, vomit continues to come out. I position the laryngoscope near the epiglottis but still can't see a thing.

"Her pulse is dropping…" the charge nurse says. I take a shot at passing the tube in the direction I think it should go. "I'm not sure I'm in, everyone start checking." I say. "I think you're in" the Respiratory Therapist says. "I'm not convinced, keep checking", I say. The oxygen saturation starts to go up however, and the pulse goes back to normal. There is good mist in the tube which comes from the lungs, and no vomit.

"Blind luck" I say out loud, and mean it. It isn't fun to try once the patient has started vomiting from previous intubation attempts, but that is how it works. And, we were all in the position of the resident at one time.

However, one thing that residents bring to the table is a nice clean slate. In the Emergency Department several years ago, a nurse checked in a patient. "Fibromyalgia, wants more narcotics", she said as she rolled her eyes. "It's her third visit here for narcotics this year."

"I'll see her" the resident said cheerfully. He immediately picked up the chart and went in the room.

"God bless him" I said to the nurse.

When he came out, about 30 minutes later, he said, "You know, I don't think this lady has fibromyalgia". I had to bite my tongue.

"OK, what do you think?"

"Well, she had been working as a professor, but about a year ago she started having chronic pain, that has never gotten better. She has been on medical leave. She always feels nauseated. It used to always be in her back but now it's in her stomach too. She's on pain meds but now they're not helping. She's lost about 30 pounds. When I examiner her, I think she may have gallstones".

I looked at him. "OK, I'll go see her, but order blood work and an ultrasound".

I go to see her. It is exactly as the resident said. The patient was a lovely woman who was on medical leave, and had been diagnosed with fibromyalgia for chronic pain symptoms. She was now on daily narcotics but felt awful all the time. She had lost weight and was often nauseated. On exam, her abdomen was tender in the right upper portion. She was taking more narcotics then she should because she was so miserable.

The ultrasound was performed in the Emergency Department, and showed a very enlarged gallbladder packed with stones, with thickening of the gallbladder wall and fluid around it. It was acutely infected, a diagnosis we call acute cholecystitis.

Ultimately, the patient had her gallbladder out, went back to work and had no more problems.

So, the patient had been incorrectly diagnosed with fibromyalgia and started on chronic narcotics. Fortunately, the resident had a nice open mind and listened carefully to the patient and examined her, and made a huge difference in her life.

These two cases summarize to me the good and bad of new physicians. Yes, you want your doctor to be experienced, but sometimes someone with an open mind and new ideas can make all the difference.

It's a Glamorous Job

I looked up to see a screaming patient, face down on a gurney, being wheeled in by paramedics. She was quite a large, 60-year-old lady, and her nightgown was hiked up above her butt. I was a little surprised that that the paramedics didn't cover her a little better. My curiously piqued, I walked in the room.

The paramedic looked at me and his look said everything about their trip in to the hospital. "She's constipated", he said. That was it. The entire report. He grabbed his chart hastily and left the room.

I spoke with the patient. She had just returned from a trip to Europe with her son and swore that she had not had a bowel movement in two weeks. Well, it could happen I guess. Two weeks is a long time.

After I examined her, I set up to disimpact her. That means I got gloves on, put a Chux (blue plastic sheets, the nurses get mad if you don't use them and get stool/blood/etc. all over the bed) under her, and put my finger up her butt.

She had a huge stool in there, the size of a very hard grapefruit. Too big to pull out but I started breaking it up with my finger. Then I could pull some of the pieces out, a slow and tedious process. She did fairly well during this actually.

After I left, the nurse brought in a commode, and in about 15 minutes she delivered a huge bowel movement that the nurse said filled the commode. I took a pass on the nurse's excited suggestion that I come look at it. Most of my coworkers were angry at me because of the way the department now smelled and they walked around with those darned peach spray bottles spraying the department, making it smell like peach and poop.

I actually have no idea who invented peach spray and I think about it often. There are no redeeming qualities to it. It comes in little white plastic hospital spray bottles, about 2 inches high. It does not smell like a peach unless it is a genetically modified chemical peach. It does not cover up smell, at all, it just adds another layer to the smell. I prefer those little glass bottles of Wintergreen that the nurses some-how find every now and then. I will hold it right under my nose and breathe that in for awhile. I do worry about what that does to my brain over the years though. Anyway, whoever invented peach spray is prob-ably very rich and all they did was make all of our lives worse.

The next day I showed up to work, and as I walked in the door no less then three people approached me to tell me I had received a gift. They all seemed quite excited. As I approached the nursing station, I saw a huge golden, shiny box of chocolates, two pounds. Everyone was anxiously awaiting for me to open it, not because they wanted me to have a gift, but because they wanted the chocolates. I slowly opened the card to make them wait. It was from the patient I disim-pacted, with a nice thank you note.

The chocolate was gone in 30 minutes, and despite the fact that I love chocolate dearly I did not have a single piece. The flashbacks of the patient's back side and her screaming as she wheeled by, the grapefruit, the disimpacted pieces of poop, and then the peach smell on top of it all was too much for me, and the chocolate didn't look so good.

That case reminds me of how unscientific our jobs in the Emer-gency Department can be. Although there are many up-to-date moni-toring systems that we have, special types of central lines, fancy ultra-sound machines and scans, and everything is computerized, a lot of times it just comes down to you and the patient and basic body func-tions. As soon as you forget that, you will miss something.

I had a patient from a motor vehicle accident who was entered into the trauma system. Being entered in the trauma system if the patient is awake brings its own trauma. Once in the trauma room, you are surrounded with multiple team members who are responsible for various functions. Your clothes are cut off within a minute or so, IV's are placed, you are on a monitor, and oxygen is placed. A complete examination is performed. The trauma surgeon and often an anesthesiologist are in attendance. This patient was a nice young man, about 20. After I did my initial portion of the exam, I put lube on my finger to do the rectal. We do this to rule assess neurologic status (rectal tone) and to check for bony fracture. I told the patient very briefly what I was going to do then quickly started the rectal.

"Wow, real high-tech job ya got there doc", the patient said. The whole trauma team laughed as did I, but the fact is, he got it exactly right. The Emergency Department all comes down to some pretty basic functions, and despite what the TV shows say there is not a lot of glamour involved.

Psychiatric Crisis

In the state where I work we have had a psychiatric crisis. Can you call it a crisis if it has gone on for more than 10 years?

About 10 years ago, one of our state's two large psychiatric hospitals was closed. It was a large hospital, but it was felt that these patients could be integrated into the community where they could be followed. The problem with that is that most of them were paranoid schizophrenics.

The majority of the time, paranoid schizophrenics do much better once they are on medication, but if left on their own often want to stop taking their medications, which is a component of the 'paranoid' part of the diagnosis. It truly is a chemical imbalance in the brain, and the medications stabilize this. They often feel that someone is trying to poison them, and they are concerned their medications are poisonous. We began seeing more and more of these chronic mentally ill in the Emergency Department at that time.

Then, we had several smaller community hospitals close their psychiatric beds for a number of reasons, one of which I am sure is that there is no money in psychiatric admissions, and our State doesn't provide adequate funding for psychiatric care. Also, bad things can happen in psychiatric hospitals, then the State will investigate and decide that there were "safety" issues, and close the unit down. Somehow it is viewed as "safer" if the patients have no where to go and no place to be cared for.

Then, our Crisis Triage Center, an outpatient clinic which handled a great many psychiatric patients, shut down due to lack of funding. I believe we pay some of the highest taxes in our state so I am not sure why that happened.

All of this has been a complete disaster for Emergency Departments in our state. These patients have nowhere to go, and either they are brought to the Emergency Department, make it there somehow on their own, or the police bring them in. Once in our Emergency Department, if it is a patient who needs acute inpatient psychiatric hospitalization, we have to wait days for beds. This fills up our Emergency Department beds, and then sick medical patients end up waiting in the lobby, then we go on Divert to ambulances (where we don't accept new medical patients by ambulance, and they have to go to other hospitals), and it just goes on and on from there.

For over ten years of this, I kept thinking it would get better, something would change, but it never has. There are often days where our Emergency Department has over 20 psychiatric patients waiting for beds in the state, some for up to a week. This is a truly horrible situation for the patients and their families.

Our nurses however have handled it with grace and incredible compassion. While Emergency Department nurses were not typically trained in long term psychiatric care, they have all done their best under dire conditions to care for these patients.

One of our charge nurses who I dearly love, Penny, has worked in the Emergency Department over 15 years. She is a very pleasant, friendly woman with beautiful short dark curly hair, purple glasses, and always with a smile. When she first came she was not very confident, and any conflict really bothered her. Since conflict is a daily part of our job, I wasn't sure if she would make it at first.

Gradually, she got more and more used to handling difficult situations. She went from being an insecure person who would actually go off by herself and cry if she had to stand up for herself, to being more and assertive. In her prior job, although I'm sure they had occasional conflicts, the conflicts probably hadn't had to be decided on the spot, without having a conference or a meeting. That can't usually happen in the Emergency Department so it takes some getting used to.

One night a psychiatric patient was put in a "psych room" (just one of the regular rooms we now use for psychiatric patients) by the police. I don't know what the charges were. When the patient was changing into a gown, the police officer stepped out of the room and closed the door. In that few minutes, the patient apparently knocked out several ceiling tiles and climbed into the metal scaffolding between our basement Emergency Department and the next floor. The police officer opened the door and realized the patient was not in there. Penney had been standing there as well and they both had stepped in the room at the same time.

They looked around the empty room, under the bed, then looked up...and saw the patient crawling away in the scaffolding. He had bashed out a lot of the ceiling squares. The police officer quickly pulled out his gun and aimed it at the patient, prepared to shoot. "STOP!!" Penny screamed. "PUT DOWN YOUR GUN.". I had made it to the room just in time to hear this. "USE YOUR TASER!" She said. Quickly the cop pulled out his Taser and tasted the patient. We all stared as the patient shook then slumped over the scaffolding.

"Great, now how do we get him out?" Penny demanded. The cop called for back up, and between several cops and our security guards got him down.

We didn't talk about this for several days, I think we were all still processing it. The next shift when I saw Penny, I wanted to tell her what a great job she did. "Well, what I wanted to scream was that there was an ICU on the very next floor, and the ICU beds are right above that area of the ER," she said. The ICU she had worked in for years was just right above us.

"When you first started here and you were so quiet and timid, I never thought you would order a cop to put down his gun", I joked. She looked shocked, then agreed with me. "No, I guess working in the ER really does change you".

Once a psychiatric facility has finally accepted a patient, we have to fill out a large packet and call report and tell them every detail of the patient. In our opinion, which may be unjust, we think they "game us", trying to delay arrival of the patient to their facility. They have to accept patients once they have a bed, but often we think the nurses at the psych hospitals want a break. Of course we might be a little jaded, and I'm sure they complain about us plenty.

One of our nurses had been watching over three very difficult psychiatric patients all night, and one of them was to be admitted to another hospital, but the hospital refused to take him until he gave a urine drug screen. He had refused to urinate in a cup the entire shift. To make matters worse, I asked this nurse every time I saw her if he had urinated yet and she was beginning to have homicidal thoughts about me. The shift progressed, no urine.

Finally, I walked out of another patient's room, and saw the nurse, bent over a large puddle on our linoleum floor, with an eye dropper. "What in the name of God are you doing?" I asked. She smiled up at me triumphantly. "Got the urine!" She said happily. The patient had walked out in the hall and peed all over the floor to keep us from getting the urine drug screen, but the nurse solved the problem. I quickly took out my iPhone and snapped her picture. The next day I thought about emailing it to the whole department as it was such a great picture but was sure that JCAHO, our governing body, would somehow find it and get the nurse in trouble, so I just printed it and left it in her mailbox, with the caption, "Only an ER nurse". She and her husband loved it.

We have a chronic psychiatric patient, Marlee, who has been in the Emergency Department over 150 times. She has schizoaffective disorder. Her modus operandi is to go to public places, take off all her clothes, and then run around. She is 6' tall and weights over 350 pounds, is amazingly strong, and it usually takes multiple police officers or security guards to take her down.

Finally, after many years, she was put in state custody, and lives in a private care home with a full time provider. She still comes in frequently. One Christmas eve she came in after they tried to take her to a movie and she went streaking through the theater. Another time she did the same at a public playground. It is not unusual while in the Emergency Department to look up and see Marlee streaking naked down the hallway, security in hot pursuit.

One night Marlee had visited the Emergency Department after telling her caregiver she was suicidal. She had stayed for some time, had stabilized, and was going home. She was just waiting for secure transport to take her back to her home. I was at the end of my shift and had changed my clothes and was leaving the Emergency Department.

Once in the parking lot, I saw a Care Car, with the security guard, Marlee's caregiver, and Penny, and clearly there was a problem. Marlee didn't want to get in the car and was being belligerent. I walked over to see if they needed help.

What I heard I will always remember. Penny stood there, in a non-confrontational stance, calmly talking with Marlee. She talked to her in a calm, soothing voice, so soft I couldn't really differentiate the words. "Do you want me to call the cops?" the security guard asked. "No, just wait a minute" Penny said, and kept calmly talking. When I arrived Marlee's face was red and blotched, but now she started looking calmer, almost sleepy. Penny continued to urge her to go home, get some rest, and watch TV. She asked what Marlee's favorite shows were. Marlee gave one word responses. Finally, after about 5 minutes, Marlee got in the car with her caregiver and they sped off.

In the Emergency Department we are always in a hurry, and patience is definitely not one of our virtues, especially not mine. Penny however spent the extra time, was compassionate to the patient, and avoided a difficult situation for everyone.

Food and Emergency Departments

No one thinks of "food" when they think of Emergency Departments, yet the subject comes up an amazing amount when you are there.

Patients are always asking for food. "When can they eat?" the family often asks. Unfortunately, every Emergency Department in the country I'm afraid has had a vending machine placed in their lobby, approved by some well-meaning administrator. I worked in a hospital once that actually had a McDonalds in the lobby. That was a big problem as patients and their families would disappear to go off and eat something.

A typical scenario runs like this. I have a five year old with an unstable elbow fracture. I see the patient, the nurse starts an IV, we get an immediate x-ray, and everything is going perfectly. I call the orthopedist to take the patient to surgery, then the immediate question, when did they last eat? As I am horrible at remembering to ask this, I run to the room, only to see the patient eating a bag of Cheet-O's. "Oh, where did those come from?" I ask, horrified.

"From the vending machine in the lobby," says the well-meaning parent. "The one with the big sign on it that says "don't eat anything until you ask your nurse or doctor?" I want to ask. Now, surgery will be delayed six hours.

I once had to transfer a patient with appendicitis to another hospital because the patient wanted a doctor who only worked there for their surgery. This was many years ago when I was new in practice. I called report and the patient left our hospital. About an hour later, I got a call from an upset surgeon because on the way, the patient's family had stopped and the patient, despite their appendicitis, wolfed down a cheeseburger. Usually patients with appendicitis absolutely will not eat or even drink because of their pain and nausea. I have to say I did not think of warning the patient and family not to go to Burger King on their way there, but since then I always give this warning.

The nursing staff are supposed to get meal breaks, but frequently they have to miss or delay them due to urgent cases. Then they have to scarf their food down in the break room, which is always dirty and the refrigerator a true health hazard. They very rarely get to eat an uninterrupted meal, even on 12 hour shifts.

We are not supposed to have food out in the Emergency Department, but there is always an emesis basin or plastic bedpan filled with jelly beans, chocolates, or the like.

My favorite surgeon every year brings in home made Baklava, which we have to put in a central area to keep everyone honest and only take one piece. It is so good I would personally sneak several pieces if it was in the break room.

Most of the physicians rarely eat on their shift unless it is a quick snack grabbed at the desk. This unfortunately often leads to feeling starved when one gets home, especially in the middle of the night.

I often wonder in other countries if they are as obsessed with eating as much as we are, and if patients frequently ask for food while in an Emergency Department for an "emergency".

Recently I took care of a very nice 70-year-old woman who was sent from a clinic because of a low heart rate. It was in the 40's. As I finished my initial questions with her, she asked me if she could eat. "No, not yet, I want to do some tests". I finished my exam and walked to the desk to order laboratories. In less than a minute, her nurse approached me.

"The lady in 37 wants to know if she can eat". I explained why I didn't want her to eat, I thought there was a possibility she might need a pacemaker and didn't want her to eat and delay a procedure.

About 10 minutes later I was performing a suture repair on another patient. "The lady in 37 wants a meal try". Same explanation.

I spoke with a cardiologist about an hour later when the tests were back. He asked for an additional study, an echocardiogram. The patient again asked to eat when I told her about the test.

The echocardiogram was normal, and I had been asked twice more if she could eat. On the final request I had given in and the nurse brought her a meal tray. We were all relieved.

When I called the cardiologist back, I told him that her pulse was 40 but all of her tests were completely normal. "Do you think she's stable enough to go home?" he asked. I thought about it, can you possibly be sick when you've asked to eat that many times? I literally based part of my clinical decision making on this.

The cardiologist saw her the next week and she was fine, and at least she wasn't hungry.

We can take care of patients...even without computers

I went to work on December 13th, and as I walked through the electronic emergency doors the department seemed OK. We never say the words "quiet" or "calm", or even think them because all Emergency Department personnel believe that is bad luck. A very superstitious bunch.

I got my scrubs on, grabbed my stethoscope and prescription pad out of my drawer, and went to work. At around 8 am, two paramedics who I know well brought in a patient who was in a motor vehicle accident, minor fender bender, but with neck pain. "It's really starting to snow out there, roads getting a little slick", they said.

I continued working, then another set of paramedics arrived a half hour later. "We're lucky to get her here", they said of the elderly woman they brought in. "It is really coming down". We live in Portland, where one inch of snow can literally close down the city. I started asking them questions about how bad it was. They told me cars were starting to slide, and have trouble getting up hills.

In Portland, we get rain for basically nine months out of the year and think nothing of it, but for our city I assume that it is cheaper to shut down the city one day a year for a bad storm rather than purchase snow removal equipment, because that is what happens. We literally shut down.

The problem here is, if it is cold enough to snow, it starts to "ice", because we've always just had rain or will get rain. If the temperature drops, the roads ice up as does everything. We have incredible ice storms that knock out power, break down incredible numbers of trees, and make driving an incredible hazard. When this happens, one of our trauma hospitals has to shut down as it is on "the Hill" in Portland, and no ambulance can get up it.

"Well, the patients are still getting here", our charge nurse said, looking at the computer. It showed many patients checking into triage with various complaints, many of which seemed storm related. Wrist pain, knee pain, back pain, most likely from falls on the ice.

"We'll be OK," I said confidently. "They will all be mild complaints".

I continued working and treating patients, when I heard an odd electrical sound, then a buzzing. Within a minute someone said the computers were down. A few seconds later we realized our phones weren't working. Apparently a car slid into our "server", shutting down everything. I have no idea where our server is but it seems like it should be in a place where a car can't hit it.

What this did to our Emergency Department was incredible. When I started working there, over 20 years ago, we had few computers and they were just for registration and what we called "Poisondex" that we could look up overdose information on. There was no internet available. I know I sound old saying that, but it really wasn't that long ago.

Hospitals joined the computer age slower than almost any company in America, probably because of concerns over confidentiality and probably because health care people are generally not good at computers in my opinion. We are all too impatient and hate new things in our established routines.

About 10 years ago, we developed our electronic medical record system, and now it is hard to believe we haven't always had it. For almost all patients, unless I have to go in the room in the first minute, I can quickly look up their records, their medications, their allergies, and even their x-rays and cardiac studies. It has changed medicine more than anything else in my career.

Prior to electronic medical records, when a patient came in, our poor secretary had to leave the department, walk down a long hall to medical records, and lug back charts, or worse, the medical records department couldn't find the chart.

Unfortunately, even though this was ten years ago, we are now so dependent on technology that we become helpless when we don't have it.

So now, the city is iced down, and our hospital's entire "server" is out. Would you not think there would be a back up server? Hopefully there is now but there sure wasn't on this day.

No medical records, no computer to look at and see where the patients were, no x-rays, just us and the patient. A moment of true panic took over for all of us.

Then the nurses started kicking in. They got out a giant white board and started writing each patients name on it. Paper charts were generated, instead of computerized. Everyone started doing whatever they could.

The biggest glitch was that the phone system was out for over an hour, but fortunately we had a back up emergency phone system which helped.

Another glitch came when we realized the hospital had NO x-ray machines that didn't run on the computer system, so we couldn't do x-rays. Everything had to be a clinical decision.

This lasted six hours. Fortunately I had all standard cases with no critical patients, and everything went pretty smoothly.

In a way, it felt good to me just to have it be me and the patient. I felt like I spent more time with each patient without all the bells and whistles. However, one of my partners described it as feeling like he was "practicing medicine underwater", because of the pace.

The computer outage lasted about six hours, and ended shortly before I went off my shift. As I walked out through the snow to my car I had never felt so tired, but I didn't have that weird amped up feeling I usually get after my shifts. I wondered if the lack of staring at a bright screen every few minutes, and instead just talking with patients, had that effect.

I'll tell you what to do

"Recurrent inflammatory gastritis", the chief complaint said on the chart I picked up. Wow, that's a pretty specific complaint. I pulled up the patient's old records on the computer before going in the room, and saw that he had prior visits and tests performed for abdominal pain over the last two years.

I walked in the room to meet him. He was sitting bolt upright in the bed, his wife in a chair next to him. "Mr. James, can you tell me about your pain?" I asked in a general way.

"I have recurrent inflammatory gastritis, and I need an IV, Protonix, Dilaudid and Zofran right now", he said. It was 2 in the morning. I stared at him dumbly. "I've never heard of that diagnosis", I said for some absolutely stupid reason. That made me sound really brilliant, and I could see he was already completely unimpressed.

"You've never heard of it?", he asked irritably. He went on to explain how two years ago while on a vacation in Hawaii he had been diagnosed with it in the Emergency Department. After coming back he had seen multiple specialists as well as his own doctor and had other testing done. He had made several visits to Emergency Department's when his pain flared up. He spoke very quickly and patronizingly to me, like I was a complete idiot. I was getting a little irritated.

"No, I've never heard about that diagnosis in my 18 years of practice," I decided to be completely honest with him; he already thought I was an idiot so we would just go with that. I had no concerns about my pride at 2 in the morning. "What tests have you had done?"

164

"Every test! I've seen every specialist. I don't need more tests, I need to get the medications I told you about. I'm in pain and I want to get going on this."

"Have you had an ultrasound?" I asked.

"I've had every test!" He almost yelled. "I've had a CAT scan, endoscopy, colonoscopy, and I've seen the best specialists for this".

"But on the charting I didn't see that you've had an ultrasound."

"I'm sure I've had an ultrasound", he said.

"Honey", his wife spoke up for the first time, "I don't remember you having an ultrasound".

"I've had every test with the best specialists, you can call my doctor," he said, getting angrier by the minute.

I had had it. "I will call him," I stated to him.

"Yes, maybe he can explain it to you, since you obviously don't know," he said.

I turned to his wife. "Does he always act like this?" I don't know what made me appeal to her, but I sensed she was an ally, I was exhausted, and this guy was treating me like shit. To my surprise, his wife actually laughed.

"Yes,", she said. "He runs a company and is used to people doing what he says".

"Well, I'll order the medicines you want, but I'm getting an ultrasound", I said. He grumpily agreed but I could see he was seething.

His blood work started coming back and was very abnormal. The ultrasound tech arrived and went in the room. About 15 minutes later I saw her leaving and caught up with her for a preliminary report. "Acute cholecystitis", she said. "Big, thick gallbladder, lots of stones, probably one in the common bile duct."

Aha! That was the reason for his intermittent pain. Gallbladder disease sometimes doesn't show up on CT scans. I was quite proud of myself.

I went in to tell him the report. I was of course very smug, but he STILL questioned my diagnosis as his "specialists" had told him the other diagnosis. Again I decided to just call it like it was.

"Well, you don't have the diagnosis they gave", I said, "They were wrong. This has absolutely been the cause of your pain, and you should be happy about it because it's a fixable problem". He looked at me, and then we actually started having a conversation. We talked about cholecystitis and the treatment.

I called the surgeon, and got him admitted. The surgeon took the gallbladder out and the patient had no complications.

Although this was a very difficult case for me, and I really don't like having interactions like this, it did bring up a good point. We can't go into cases with a closed mind. We have to have an open mind. The easiest thing would have been to just go along with this Type A guy and do what he wants, but that can lead to disaster. Some smart patients try to tell you what to do, and sometimes that is fine, but you still have to do the exact same job with everyone.

One of my partners, who I think the world of, took care of an elderly lady many years ago in our department, the wife of a retired physician. The patient was on Coumadin, a blood thinner, and had fallen and hit her head. She had a laceration that needed repaired also.

My partner wanted to order a CT scan, which we usually do if the patient is on Coumadin, but the husband didn't think she needed it, and declined. That patient went home and died of a brain hemorrhage. Everyone was devastated.

It just brings up the point, you have to pull the proverbial trigger in the Emergency Department, and always suspect the worse possible case. Yeah, we radiate too many patients with CT's, but I have never regretted getting a CT and I have regretted not getting a CT. The bottom line is, we don't know the patient, we don't know their pain threshold, we don't know their personality or background, and we have one shot at them. If they didn't have a serious problem they wouldn't have come to the Emergency Department, they would have gone to a doctors office or not come in (OK, we all know that isn't completely true, but you just have to go with that one).

When you treat everyone from homeless people to extremely wealthy people, from IV drug abusers to celebrities, from nursing home patients to NBA players, you need to remember that it all comes down to assessing the situation and making a diagnosis. That is it. Although they are all different and have different needs, you need to listen to the cues that are all around you and error on the side of caution in every case.

Altered Level of Consciousness

Everyone wonders, when they hear of a mistake made in the Emergency Department, how that could ever happen. I've been at dinner parties where someone knew someone who went to the Emergency Department and was misdiagnosed, and everyone expresses shock and disappointment.

One time on a plane I read a USA Today story about a doctor in an Emergency Department who missed a myocardial infarction (heart attack) in an elderly male patient. I don't remember now why this had become a news story. "Wow," I thought, "that happens in every Emergency Department in this country!" Believe it or not, patients having myocardial infarctions come in with a bizarre array of symptoms, not always the classic chest pain down the left arm, and some people have no pain at all.

Plus, the medical tests are not perfect (by a long shot) to make the diagnosis. Even EKG's are off the mark about 50% of the time! The USA Today article was shocked that this diagnosis got missed on this patient.

I, on the other hand, wonder how we make the correct diagnosis as often as we do. I'm always surprised we don't screw things up way more often to be completely honest. Patients have symptoms that aren't typical, we get half the story, we don't have their old records because their doctors office is closed, their own doctor isn't on call so we can't find out their history, they left out the part that they used cocaine last night or that they had just been admitted to another hospital for the same complaint , the list goes on and on .

This week I took care of a 35-year-old patient brought in by paramedics for "vaginal bleeding and painful cramps". I heard the nurse

168

grumbling about taking an ambulance for your period. I went to take report from the paramedics. The patient, who was Vietnamese speaking mainly, had her period start 3 days ago. She had a history of a tubal ligation. She always took herbal tea for her period but it was much worse, so she took more tea than usual. She had never had vaginal bleeding like this.

She was very tender across her entire abdomen. I immediately wondered about tubal pregnancy, which can happen after tubal ligation, and ordered a stat pregnancy test and an ultrasound. We gave her IV fluids as her blood pressure was low.

The pregnancy test came back quickly and was negative. I went back in; now a cousin was there who could interpret for us. The patient kept describing her period, how awful it was. She had drunk the herbal tea. "How much?" I asked. "Six cups in one hour". The cousin fortunately had brought in the tea. I called Poison Center. The tea was a mixture of senna and peppermint oil, the Poison Center nurse told me. "It could definitely cause severe abdominal pain and cramping". Ahh, I thought happily, there is our diagnosis.

Then, her blood work came back. Her White Blood Cell count was quite high. I went back in and examined the patient. She had such a tender abdomen. "Screw it", I thought, scientifically-like, "I'm ordering a CT scan". I ordered the CT to put my mind at rest. I cancelled the ultrasound.

An hour later the radiologist called, "Ruptured appy, lots of bowel contents everywhere, real disaster", he said.

I was shocked. From vaginal bleeding, to calling Poison Center, to a ruptured appendix? If we had missed that diagnosis and sent her home she could have died. It was especially unusual because she didn't have any vomiting at all which usually accompanies appendicitis, she could easily drink fluids which is atypical, and her pain wasn't worse on the right.

Another patient, about a 30-year-old woman, came in with severe abdominal cramping and diarrhea. After I did a huge workup, I told her that her intestines looked very abnormal on CT scan, and that her blood work was very abnormal, but that I couldn't figure out exactly what was wrong with her. She then admitted she had been taking a supplement she bought from her hairdresser. She hadn't told me about it initially.

A quick call to Poison Center revealed that it was actually algae-type scum taken off of Klamath Falls, a large body of water in Oregon that is more like a lake. It was marketed originally as a diet aide I believe. It had been pulled from the market but somehow a few bottles survived. She was quite sick and had to be admitted; initially I had thought she would have to go to surgery so this piece of information made a big difference.

In my first year of practice I took care of a lovely young woman, who was non-English speaking. She was brought to my area because "they wanted a woman doctor". The family and the patient also refused to have her change into our hospital gown for reasons of modesty.

The patient was there for vomiting. Her husband interpreted. "She is just vomiting, vomiting", he kept saying. "You need to give her medicine to make her quit vomiting". "Does she have a headache?" I asked, several times, and was told no. We gave her IV fluids and IV nausea medications. She kept intermittently vomiting. Her labs and pregnancy test were normal. Her stomach didn't hurt. Her urine was normal. Finally I re-examined her. Her left pupil was very dilated. Had it been like that when I first examined her? But she was still alert which didn't make sense. I ordered a stat CT of her brain.

To my surprise, she had a hemorrhage right at a portion of her brain that is involved with the nerves to the eye, which had caused it to look abnormal on one side. She had a blown pupil because of that, very rare.

By this time, a woman friend of the patient's arrived in the room. This was in the days before we had translators widely available. When I asked her to ask the patient if she had a headache, the patient described a severe, splitting headache. The husband had told me no headache three times.

I learned from this case to not just listen to the family and not let the family translate. They may have their own agenda or may not be good translators. Her husband was in a big rush to get her better and take her home, I think because they had a baby at home that needed her care.

Often things in the Emergency Department are not straight forward to say the least. A little detective work can be fun, but when I think back on cases like these I just feel lucky and relieved that the diagnosis was picked up, sometimes in spite of us.

Brothers and Sisters

I would estimate that out of all the pediatric patients I take care of, approximately 1 or 2 percent are there because of trauma inflicted by their dear brothers and sisters. Nothing malicious, just typical things that happen in every family. My own husband has scars left from trauma inflicted by his two older brothers, with some pretty scary stories to go with them.

The typical is a push or shove, someone's head goes into a dresser, or they get pushed from a bunk bed. Someone goes flying off the trampoline at the hands of their older sister, or in a fit of anger the brother throws a can of soup at an annoying older sib. Some are completely accidental; I bet I have had 10 patients over the years with significant injuries from standing too near their brother while he was practicing batting or golfing. The parents are always very upset but it is pretty standard stuff.

A baby that I took care of years ago came in with a complaint of "choking". I watched the mom carry it down the hall; it was smiling and cooing, about 4 months old. I went in to ask her what was going on; the baby looked fantastic.

"When I lay him down he starts choking", she explained. She said he had had a small cold and cough, but no fever. I carefully examined him while he was in mom's arms, and ordered an x-ray to rule out pneumonia.

I promptly moved on to the next patient, when I heard "Code Blue, x-ray". X-ray has many rooms so it never crossed my mind that it would be this baby. However, when I showed up it was this baby, but mom was holding him and he looked fantastic. "When I laid him down to set up the machine, he stopped breathing and turned blue!" The

172

frantic x-ray tech said. I cancelled the x-ray and we rushed him back to the Emergency Department. My older, wiser partner suggested we get set up for emergent intubation and then lay the baby down.

By now, we had 3 nurses, a tech, and two doctors ready for the intubation. Medications were drawn up, the baby was on a monitor and pulse ox, and we had our equipment ready.

We had mom lay the perfectly normal appearing baby down. He immediately started turning blue, amazing. I quickly looked into his throat to intubate him. To my surprise, I was met with a large piece of metal. "I see something metal…" I said to the team. My partner quickly handed me a special forceps that we use for removal of foreign bodies, called a Magill's forceps, and I gently pulled it out. My next thought was to go ahead and intubate because my adrenaline was up, but my partner suggested waiting a few minutes. As always he was right and after the giant wing-nut was removed the baby was breathing completely normally, even when lying down.

We all then stood, shocked, staring at the happy baby. The mom was in complete disbelief at the giant wing-nut, now lying on a tray.

She pieced it together for us. The family was going through a huge re-model. They tried to keep the kids away from everything, but the older brother loved "feeding the baby", and she figured he had found the wing-nut in the construction mess and had "fed" it to the baby. This could have been a true catastrophe, but thank God everything fell into place, and the mom recognized that something was very wrong.

At the other end of the spectrum, I often think of three brothers that I saw several years ago. Two of the brothers brought in their older brother, who felt like he was having a rapid heart rate. The triage nurse brought him right back.

"It's probably nothing", said the young man, who was about 25. His two brothers started helping him out of the wheelchair that the nurse insisted that he come back in. "I've had it before, and I've seen a cardiologist, but nothing ever shows up". The tech rapidly placed the monitor leads on his chest, and I glanced at the monitor.

His brothers explained that the patient had not wanted to come in, because every time he was seen with this rapid heart rate, nothing ever showed up on the monitor. So they had loaded him in the car and forced him to come to the Emergency Department.

It looked to me like a common rhythm that we see, PSVT (paroxysmal supraventricular tachycardia), but my first thought was that there was something slightly different about it than the usual. We rapidly got an EKG while I asked him questions. He had started having this several years ago, and it made him feel lightheaded, but it usually didn't last that long. He had seen his own doctor, who sent him to the cardiologist. It had never lasted this long. He was going about 170 on the monitor now.

I decided to proceed with adenosine, a medicine we usually use for PSVT. This is a medicine we give rapid IV push thru a large IV, and it typically converts PSVT back to normal "sinus" rhythm. But because something just seemed not right to me, I asked the nurse to hook him up to the pads and defibrillator in case we needed to "shock" or cardiovert him. There was just something a little odd about the configuration of the rhythm. The medicine I planned to give, adenosine, makes the patient feel odd for a minute or so and I warned him of that. His brothers sat silently the whole time as I explained everything. I asked if they wanted to stay in the room and they both nodded calmly.

The nurse rapidly administered the adenosine, 6 mg IV. As I watched the monitor, instead of going down, his heart rate shot up to 240. His blood pressure, which had been normal, dropped to 80/p. He was already hooked to the pads, and we rapidly sedated him. I asked the nurse to charge the defibrillator and set it to "synch", and we cardioverted him at 100 Joules.

Several nurses and techs were now in the room to help as they had seen there was a problem. I warned the brothers quickly what it would look like when their brother was shocked. "Clear!" the nurse said and the patient was shocked.

No change, still pulse of 240. We rapidly re-charge the machine and shocked him at 200 Joules. "Clear!" I looked at the monitor. No change, actually up to about 250, the rhythm racing across the screen. "Don't even re-check his blood pressure, just go to 300" I said to the nurse. His brothers said not a word, just sat there quietly, they didn't even look upset.

"Clear!" The nurse said. The patient's body jerked with the repeat shock. I stared at the monitor as the rhythm suddenly converted to normal "sinus" rhythm. The nurse and I took a deep breath, then she immediately went back to work checking the patient's vital signs and blood pressure. Mine and the nurse's blood pressure slowly returned to normal. I looked at the sleeping patient. He was out from the medications, but had normal vital signs now. I turned to the brothers, who still sat calmly, as if nothing had happened.

"Well, that was not how this usually goes..." I started, and explained to them that the medicine had not worked for him; I felt he had some type of atypical dysrhythmia, and explained why we had to go to rapidly shocking him electrically three times. They nodded, agreeing calmly with everything I said. They were so young, and handled it so well and so calmly, I was very impressed. None of the brothers had to be more than 26 or 26 years old I guessed. It was a lucky thing they had had the foresight to force their brother to come to the Emergency Department.

We got another EKG that showed it was normal, but I knew that he had to have some type of abnormal re-entrant electrical pathway in his heart, and I consulted the cardiologist.

After I got off the phone, I was walking back to the room, to talk to the now awake patient. .As I approached, I heard his brothers talking to him.

"Dude, it was so cool. She gave you medicine then you were out in like, one second. Then they like, electrocuted you like in the movies. Zap! Your whole body jumped off the bed", his brother explained it. The two brothers explained it to him, as they went thru the three shocks, explaining it graphically to their brother. The two brothers laughed nervously as they explained it to the patient. This was typical brotherly behavior, but I was very impressed with how they had acted in the room during a very stressful event.

The patient was admitted and taken to the electrophysiology laboratory, where he was found to have an underlying abnormal electrical system and was "ablated", meaning they electrically destroyed the extra electrical area that was causing this problem, and he did well and went home.

I think I know what I have...

On the other hand, I've had patients tell me what they have and have saved me a lot of work.

One patient came in just for weakness. She looked fine to me; she was about 35, tan, thin. She wanted a workup for the weakness. I took a complete history and was a little stumped. I was thinking in my head, well, I could order a chemistry panel to see if her electrolytes are off, a complete blood count, I guess urine...

Finally I just asked her, "what do YOU think is going on"? She was a very polite person, and paused. "Well, I think I have adrenal insufficiency", she said quietly. I stared at her. This is a very rare diagnosis, certainly not one made in Emergency Departments. "Why do you think you have that?" In my mind, I had already wondered if she had been reading too much on the internet, which does happen.

"Well, my sister had it, and I have the exact same symptoms. I feel so weak, and I've gotten really tan".

This is not a test we do in the Emergency Department typically, but I called the internal medicine consultant and discussed it. We ordered a chemistry panel, which showed that her potassium was very elevated, and her sodium decreased, hallmarks of adrenal insufficiency. Then we ordered a special test, one that I vaguely remembered from my medical school days, which was an initial blood test to look for adrenal insufficiency, and it was positive.

When my partners found out I diagnosed adrenal insufficiency in the Emergency Department, they were very impressed, but I had to 'fess up and tell them that the patient diagnosed it herself.

The other side of this occurs too. I had a very pleasant father come in with a lovely 2 month old infant. He had been watching her sleep, and noticed her irregular breathing pattern. He then had gone to the internet and researched breathing disorders. He actually found videos on some of them, showing patients with severe obstructive sleep apnea, severe Cheyne Stokes respirations, and the like. He had me watch all of them as he had actually brought them in on his video camera, and then wanted me to explain why his daughter didn't have those diseases, which I did. All the while the baby slept peacefully near us, with her normal irregular breathing pattern that all infants have. At the end of our visit he seemed satisfied and agreed to follow up with his pediatrician. Well, at least the baby has a dad who really cares about her, plus he will probably be a big help when it is time for her first big research paper some day.

Once when working with a resident, he described to me a patient he had just seen, a 55-year-old woman, who had chest pain. Her EKG and chest x-ray were completely normal when I reviewed them. I went in and sat down and spoke with her. She was extremely worried about her chest pain, and described it in detail. It would come on, last just a few minutes, then leave, then in 15 minutes come back.

Her pain wasn't related to activity or rest, and wasn't related to food. She had noticed it over the last few days, but it was much worse today. She had not felt "right" though for several months, and had thought that her chest felt "funny". She wasn't short of breath, and she didn't have a fever or cough.

None of her symptoms made sense to me or fit into any "classic" patterns. Finally I asked her, "What is it that you are concerned about? What do you think you have?'

"Well", she answered, "I think I have the same thing John Ritter had".

I was very shocked that she said this. John Ritter had a dissecting thoracic aneurysm. I should have asked her where she read this or how she knew about it, as I don't think the average person knew that much about his medical issues, but her answer was good enough for me. I ordered a chest CT scan with contrast.

About 30 minutes later the radiologist called me, and methodically described her chest CT. "Normal lungs, no pulmonary embolus," he started.

"OK, thanks" I said, thinking he was done with his report.

"But, she does have a very large aortic aneurysm, and there is one part that I am worried about that may be dissecting". Her thoracic aorta was increased at 6 cm, normal is 2.

I admitted her to the ICU, and did tell the cardiothoracic surgeon how I diagnosed it. He couldn't believe it.

Many patients are amazingly smart, and people today are just better read and really knowledgeable about medical care.

Unsolicited Advice

I have taken care of thousands of patients over the years, and I have advice if you ever visit the Emergency Department (hopefully you never have to).

Try to keep a list of your health problems, medications, and allergies and carry it with you in your wallet or enter the information in your cell phone. Even though you can name them all right now, when you are sick you may not be able to. Also if you have elderly parents, they should carry the same information with them at all times.

It is obviously not a good day for you if you are in the Emergency Department, and we know that. But please be as nice as possible to the nurses. If you have a complaint about one, do it a few days later to an administrator, but it won't help to start yelling at them. I'm sure you can imagine how much abuse they put up with on a daily basis. They can be your best friend throughout the process in the Emergency Department, trust me on that.

If, God forbid, your kid has to come to the Emergency Department, bring something for them such as a blanket or favorite stuffed animal if they are small, and books if there is a wait and it isn't a huge emergency. If they are older, hand-held video games or cell phone games are very helpful (yes, it is a lie that cell phones disrupt the monitors, we just don't like them).

Be completely honest with all of the staff, and include small things that may help them. List all of your medications truthfully including the herbal ones; a lot of us use herbal medications too, and no one will think it is weird. It can be really important. A lot of people won't tell about medications like Viagra, and this can have severe complications if we give nitro for angina.

One big complaint we hear, is "the last person just asked me that". We frequently ask the same questions over and over, and it is amazing how much the story changes each time. The reason for that is simple: Patient's are sick, and often scared, when they come in. It happens ten times a shift that the patient will tell the nurse they only take Metoprolol, and that they have no medical problems. This goes on the chart. When the nurse in the room asks, they remember that they also take a baby aspirin a day, this is important. Then when I see them they tell me that they do have a history of high blood pressure, but didn't list it because they consider it under control on medication. This makes perfect sense, but is the reason we keep asking. Sometimes the patient will remember something they hadn't thought of earlier.

List your family members under "ICE" (In Case of Emergency) on your cell phone, or carry it on a card in your wallet. This has made a huge difference in critical cases. It is horrible to not be able to reach a family member of a critical patient for hours because we have no contact information at all. If you run/jog/walk/bike without a wallet, consider keeping this information in a wrist band or pocket when you are out. I have used patient's cell phone many, many times to contact family members, and having the most important call you want us to make in one spot is very helpful.

Most importantly, do not hesitate to tell any information that you think may be even remotely relevant ("Do you think it could be food poisoning? I ate at a buffet last night", or "I just started a new powdered diet program, do you think it could be related") . And never hesitate to ask questions. No one in the Emergency Department will be afraid of your questions, and we would rather have you ask them. The Emergency Department nurse often has 3-4 patients, and the doctor may have 7, 8, depending on the Emergency Department, even up to 12 or even more at a time. Checking on things and asking questions will only help, trust me on that one.

Hopefully you will never need to visit an Emergency Department, but you should know that everyone who works there is there because they want to be, and even if they seem hurried or gruff, they are there to help you in any way they can.

Made in the USA
Lexington, KY
18 October 2011